DECOLONIZING

T0270537

Unsettling Conversations about
Social Research Methods

Jacqueline M. Quinless

Decolonizing Data explores how ongoing structures of colonialization negatively impact the well-being of Indigenous peoples and communities across Canada, resulting in persistent health inequalities. In addressing the social dimensions of health, particularly as they affect Indigenous peoples and BIPOC communities, *Decolonizing Data* asks, Should these groups be given priority for future health policy considerations?

Decolonizing Data provides a deeper understanding of the social dimensions of health as applied to Indigenous peoples, who have been historically underfunded in and excluded from health services, programs, and quality of care; this inequality has most recently been seen during the COVID-19 pandemic.

Drawing on both western and Indigenous methodologies, this unique scholarly contribution takes both a sociological perspective and the "two-eyed seeing" approach to research methods. By looking at the ways that everyday research practices contribute to the colonization of health outcomes for Indigenous peoples, *Decolonizing Data* exposes the social dimensions of healthcare and offers a careful and respectful reflection on how to "unsettle conversations" about applied social research initiatives for our most vulnerable groups.

JACQUELINE M. QUINLESS is an adjunct professor in the Department of Sociology at the University of Victoria.

DECOLONIZING DATA

UNSETTLING CONVERSATIONS
ABOUT SOCIAL RESEARCH METHODS

JACQUELINE M. QUINLESS

UNIVERSITY OF TORONTO PRESS
Toronto Buffalo London

ISBN 978-1-4875-0440-3 (cloth)   ISBN 978-1-4875-3010-5 (EPUB)
ISBN 978-1-4875-2333-6 (paper)   ISBN 978-1-4875-3009-9 (PDF)

Library and Archives Canada Cataloguing in Publication

Title: Decolonizing data : unsettling conversations about social research
methods / Jacqueline M. Quinless.
Names: Quinless, Jacqueline M., author.
Description: Includes bibliographical references and index.
Identifiers: Canadiana (print) 2021035187X | Canadiana (ebook)
20210352000 | ISBN 9781487523336 (paper) | ISBN 9781487504403 (cloth) |
ISBN 9781487530105 (EPUB) | ISBN 9781487530099 (PDF)
Subjects: LCSH: Social sciences – Research – Canada. |
LCSH: Indigenous peoples – Health and hygiene – Canada. |
LCSH: Decolonization – Canada.
Classification: LCC H62.5.C3 Q56 2022 | DDC 300.72/071 – dc23

We wish to acknowledge the land on which the University of Toronto Press
operates. This land is the traditional territory of the Wendat, the Anishnaabeg,
the Haudenosaunee, the Métis, and the Mississaugas of the Credit First
Nation.

University of Toronto Press acknowledges the financial support of the
Government of Canada, the Canada Council for the Arts, and the Ontario Arts
Council, an agency of the Government of Ontario, for its publishing activities.

Canada Council   Conseil des Arts
for the Arts   du Canada

ONTARIO ARTS COUNCIL
CONSEIL DES ARTS DE L'ONTARIO
an Ontario government agency
un organisme du gouvernement de l'Ontario

Funded by the   Financé par le
Government   gouvernement
of Canada   du Canada

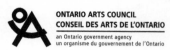

I dedicate this book to my children
and to Indigenous peoples and Researchers working
with Indigenous peoples.

Contents

Figures and Tables

Figures

Tables

Preface

Since the onset of 2020 we have been confronted by COVID-19, a global pandemic that continues to evolve at an accelerated pace in all countries around the world. According to the World Health Organization, COVID-19 is a viral infectious disease of the coronavirus family that was discovered when an outbreak began in Wuhan, China, in December 2019 (WHO, 2020). There is no doubt that we are living in a time that is rife with uncertainty, social distancing, isolation, and fear and there is a critical need to understand how the social determinants of health have an impact on individuals as well as whole communities and nations. José Francisco Cali Tzay (Guatemala), Special Rapporteur on the rights of Indigenous peoples for the United Nations Human Rights Office of the High Commissioner (2020), warns of the impact of COVID-19 on Indigenous peoples worldwide. Indigenous peoples in Canada already have high rates of chronic health conditions such as diabetes and hypertension that, coupled with social factors such as climate change, systemic racism, discrimination, and poverty, could heighten the risk of COVID-19 for many Indigenous peoples.

Canada has a colonial history that has had a devastating impact on Indigenous peoples and I believe that amid COVID-19, addressing the social dimensions of health should be ranked high among priorities for future health policy considerations. This book is part of a COVID-19 ready scholarly response that focuses on gaining a deeper understanding of the social dimensions of health as applied to Indigenous peoples who have been historically underfunded and excluded when it comes to health services, programs, and quality of care. The social dimensions of health, especially during a global pandemic, should indeed also be part of academic institutional responses to working with and supporting Indigenous research initiatives.

Since the final report of the Truth and Reconciliation Commission (TRC) in 2015, the Indigenization of Canadian universities has been high among priorities set by university administration offices. Many post-secondary institutions across the country are now sharing their strategic priorities regarding their Indigenous plans, territorial acknowledgments, and active Indigenous hiring and are striking task forces and committees. Post-secondary institutions across Canada and major funding agencies such as the Social Science and Humanities Research Council (SSHRC), Canadian Institutes of Health Research (CIHR), and Natural Sciences and Engineering Research Council (NSERC) have been responding in various ways to address the TRC's ninety-four multifaceted Calls to Action. One Call to Action in particular, number sixty-five, is worth noting:

> We call upon the federal government, through the Social Sciences and Humanities Research Council, and in collaboration with Aboriginal peoples, post-secondary institutions and educators, and the National Centre for Truth and Reconciliation and its partner institutions, to establish a national research program with multi-year funding to advance understanding of reconciliation. (TRC, 2015, p. 242)

In the past several years, Canadian universities and colleges have been moving forward with research protocols. As well, the SSHRC has summarized how it intends to fund Indigenous research through SSHRC initiatives to support Indigenous research and talent as well as upcoming SSHRC Knowledge Synthesis Grants about Indigenous peoples' reconciliation (SSHRC, 2016). In fact, Ted Hewitt, president of the SSHRC, has held the position that "social science and humanities scholars and their partners across the country are in a position to facilitate access to knowledge in all of these areas – knowledge properly grounded in relations of respect, diversity and reciprocity between Indigenous and academic communities" (Hewitt, 2016, p. 1). There is currently considerable interest inside and outside the academy in a range of issues associated with decolonizing research methods and Indigenizing health research. Part of the challenge is that the link between the ninety-four Calls to Action of the TRC and research work, especially among non-Indigenous researchers, is still not clear. Indigenous peoples and communities have long experienced exploitation by researchers and to counter that there is increasing focus on participatory action research and decolonizing research processes (Smith, 2006, 2012). As researchers, we must consider that our research practices and outcomes are "affiliated with mainstream institutions – and irrespective of our personal commitments and intentions – we are located at a nexus of power in the dominant society" (Menzies, 2001, p. 22). This means that applied research methodologies should not remain inaccessible to the people and communities we work with in generating knowledge and outcomes.

As a settler-ally and a sociologist, I have been reflecting on what this means for our research and pedagogical practices and for student learning and how we can better focus our attention on Indigenization and decolonization. I do not think I am alone when I ask, "As a non-Indigenous scholar, how does one move forward with decolonization of research practices and where should I begin?" I wrote this book as a unique scholarly contribution for other researchers, practitioners, and graduate students who may be pondering similar questions about Indigenization and decolonization of their research work. In doing so, I offer a careful and respectful reflection based in many years of my own research experience with Indigenous communities and organizations on how to "unsettle conversations" about research.

The central argument of this book is that state-centric colonial structures exert a form of structural violence on Indigenous peoples because they exercise colonial power over them by legitimizing western ways of thinking about well-being over Indigenous ways of "being well." This argument is based in evidence-supported research findings. If non-Indigenous researchers are to understand and address health inequalities that exist today for Indigenous peoples, then I suggest that careful consideration is needed about how the ways in which we teach our research practices to students and apply them as practitioners support a colonial way of thinking about and doing social research. We must ask ourselves if what we are doing is derived from colonial praxis. This book is an invitation for non-Indigenous researchers to look at the ways in which everyday research practices, particularly within the social sciences, contribute to the colonization of research practices and data. These practices have caused and continue to cause harm for Indigenous peoples. Non-Indigenous scholars need to start to look at doing research in different ways, which means that this conversation will most likely be uncomfortable for many people but it is through this discomfort that we will gather valuable insights into respect and relational accountability as pathways that open space for Indigenization. I have come to understand that Indigenization is about infusing the academy with Indigenous knowledge and applying decolonial practices through our research work to strip away the colonial knowledge systems and institutions that prevent Indigenous knowledge from flourishing.

Relational Accountability

I am a second-generation immigrant, which means, like the majority of people, a settler on Turtle Island (an Indigenous name for the continent also known as North America). I am an ethnically blended and biracial person of mixed European (Irish/ British) and Indian ancestry. My father, grandparents, and ancestors are from the communities of Secunderabad and Hyderabad in central India and, although my father settled on Turtle Island in 1967, several of my relatives still live throughout India. My personal journey of cultural diversity reads more as a story of paradox. At times, I embrace a rich sense of cultural awareness and at other times I suffer from my family's assimilation processes after their arrival to Canada, including dispossession from their native Hindi language, traditions, and customary clothing and adherence to the anglo-conformity model of mainstream western culture. It seems to me that dominant society has played an instrumental role in telling us who we are and how we should recognize and express our Indian identity. Throughout much of my life, I have internalized racism and negative stereotypes and know what it feels like to be silenced and have social worth assigned by others based on skin colour and ethnic origins. As a blended person, my identity is not inseparable from these experiences but emerges from an intersection of structures of oppression such as my gender, family origins, skin colour, and the tensions experienced through a relational process with various social institutions and other groups along the way.

I feel accountable to my research relationships and the types of research work I have been doing for nearly two decades. I started my research career fresh out of my undergraduate degree in sociology in my first job as a research assistant working at the Population Research Lab at the University of Alberta, and a few years later was delighted to become employed as a researcher and course instructor at Statistics Canada. At this time, I was 25 years old and eager to learn as much as possible about "how to" do good research. It seemed that I was well positioned to learn everything there was to know about all aspects of research design processes, applying mixed methods research, and working with diverse groups of people. This combined academic-government environment seemed like a dream come true for an aspiring early-career researcher at 25 years old because it offered many training opportunities and appeared to me at the time to be an optimal learning ground. During my tenure (1998 to 2008) with the federal government, I designed and created research courses, managed research services, and collaborated on projects with other key stakeholders in other government departments, academia, and private industry on major research initiatives such as the Data Liberation Initiative, the Education Liaison Program, the Census of Population, and the Gathering Strength Initiative for the Royal Commission on Aboriginal Peoples. In 2000 and again in 2004 I was awarded the Statistics Canada Employee Recognition Award from the Assistant Chief Statistician of Canada for an exceptional and distinguished contribution to the effectiveness of Statistics Canada. I was developing a reputation for myself as a good researcher and gaining accolades within and outside the organization. As a member of the Gathering Strength Initiative I worked in numerous Indigenous communities, teaching people about research design, mostly from a quantitative perspective. I was also involved in Census data collection activities, hiring and managing research teams comprised of hundreds of First Nations staff throughout BC coastal communities, Vancouver Island, and Northern Canada. This journey offered considerable teachings about the myriad of ways of doing good as well as bad research with Indigenous communities. Although I am no longer employed with Statistics Canada, I have been invited to join statistical technical advisory committees for input into shaping existing and emerging survey instruments, to co-chair national Indigenous data conferences, and to manage large-scale data collection operations such as the 2011 Census and National Household Survey.

Since my days as a public servant, my career has shifted and changed considerably and I am thankful for the long-lasting friendships with many colleagues. Much of my research and scholarly work now focuses on working directly with Indigenous peoples, communities, and organizations to co-create knowledge on a diverse range of issues, such as addressing children's wellness outcomes; advocating for traditional knowledge practice; addressing gendered violence resulting from industrial camps (extractive industries) in the resource development sector in British Columbia that results from a lack of anti-racist, anti-colonial employee training programs and from normalized stereotypes about Indigenous peoples; and addressing gendered violence more generally. My work with Indigenous peoples in Canada has always been based in friendships and familial bonds well established over two decades of work, which has brought me to the writing of this book. I have often wondered why I have felt such ease working with Indigenous peoples in Canada and other nations around the globe. I have been curious about the parallels this may have to my own Indian ancestry and ethnicity with shared experiences of dispossession, forced relocation, and colonialism and the resultant trauma from these experiences that have directly impacted me and my family. I believe that this has been formative in shaping my identity and my relationships with Indigenous peoples.

About This Book

This book is not about Indigenous methodologies; there are many good sources in this area written by qualified scholars and practitioners (Absolon, 2011; Kovach, 2005, 2009; Iwama et al., 2009; Smith, 1999; Wilson, 2008). Rather, this book offers a conversation about how ongoing structures of colonialization negatively impact the well-being of Indigenous peoples and communities across Canada that has resulted in persistent health inequalities. This book is a unique scholarly contribution that yields valuable insights into addressing health inequalities and intends to bring the concept of decolonizing research methods and Indigenous peoples into mainstream sociology in a way that has until now been neglected. For me, the decolonization of research within social sciences is about relational allyship, partnership, honouring Indigenous ethical protocols, holding space for resurgence, and challenging power structures. In decolonizing my own research praxis, I have reflected about the power structures that define and uphold my thoughts and practices. I explain how research design practices need to be culturally responsive, which means that researchers need to work in partnership with Indigenous peoples, communities, and/or organizations in such a way as to avoid misinterpretations and misrepresentations in the knowledge inquiry process. These are partnerships that will facilitate meaningful dialogue because Indigenous peoples, communities, and organizations can re-story the historical trauma on a number of levels to recreate new ways of understanding and contesting the deeply ingrained structures of inequality.

How the Book Is Organized

This book is organized into six chapters. Chapter one is the introduction and situates the book's topic within a broader range of contemporary concerns over the relation among settler relations in Canada, ongoing colonial practices, and Indigenous health and wellness in Canada. I argue that critical reflection on research methodologies has something important to add to these issues and I offer solutions that centre Indigenous knowledge systems to address health inequalities.

Chapter two provides a critical review of the impacts of colonization on Indigenous peoples in Canada. The discussion focuses on government assimilation policy, the reserve system, and residential schools and outlines the effects of colonization in the context of health and well-being. The chapter discusses the 2015 Truth and Reconciliation Commission and the ninety-four Calls to Action and how they are related to health and well-being but that little has been accomplished since 2015. A central theme of this chapter is the ongoing processes of colonialism through the legacies of the residential school system, Indian Act, Department of Indian Affairs, and ongoing state-centric colonial practices, which all have negative impacts on different states of Indigenous well-being. Chapter three explores health and wellness and struggles for self-determination coupled with a holistic understanding of health and wellness that relies on the First Nations Perspective on Health and Wellness (FNPOW) and the interrelationship and balance between physical, mental, emotional, and spiritual aspects of the Traditional Medicine Wheel (FNHA, 2013a). This provides a contextual understanding of how Indigenous peoples' relationship to colonialism has impacted overall states of health and wellness. Given that little substantive research has examined the complexities of urban Indigenous health and wellness using participatory action research that incorporates a mixed-methods approach, this chapter makes an important contribution to the urban Indigenous health literature by examining the role that FNPOW plays in shaping holistic health.

The concept of social capital first articulated by Pierre Bourdieu provided an initial theoretical framework, which has been further developed by studies of well-being. Social capital has been well identified in the literature as an important resource for community capacity building and for fostering the good life in an urban context (Gray et al., 2008; Hill & Cooke, 2014; Newhouse & Fitzmaurice, 2012; Simpson, 2011). Chapter four on social capital and strategies for building community capacity reviews the conceptual frameworks and measurement tools that have been developed since the 1970s by various countries, organizations, and groups as composite measures of well-being. The link between social capital analysis and Indigenous well-being is important when we examine the state-centric approaches through frameworks and indicators that have been developed to measure Indigenous wellness and its associated attributes in Canada. Empirical research into the association between social capital and health has provided strong support for considering social capital as a health determinant, with testable hypotheses and interpretive results (Robson & Sanders, 2009). This chapter considers the relationships that occur across individual and community levels of well-being that emerge in the urban landscape and how social capital can be applied to health and wellness within urban Indigenous communities.

Chapter five on two-eyed seeing and decolonizing research methods will show that participatory action research differs from most other approaches to Indigenous health and wellness research. The conversation will describe how participatory action research, using mixed methods, creates openings for reflection, knowledge co-creation, and action that aim to improve health and reduce health inequities through involving the people who, in turn, take actions to improve their own health (Castellano, 2004; Smith, 1999). In this chapter I explain how to create a study that demonstrates the extent to which both Indigenous and western knowledge can be reconciled while at the same time maintaining academic rigour and supporting a two-eyed way of seeing health and wellness.

Chapter six, the concluding chapter, will bring together the themes discussed in the previous chapters and will discuss the importance of honouring Indigenous ethical protocols, the limitations of the two-eyed seeing approach, and allyship through responsive research. In doing so, the chapter will bring together many concepts, such as self-determination, decolonization, and research methods and situate the conversation in the context of social capital analysis in relation to Indigenous health and well-being as we go forward. The discussion will also show how these concepts relate to a critical engagement of social research methods with the introduction of an innovative and integrative methodology of participatory action research, which we refer to as responsive research and the Translocal relationships, Responsibility to partners, Accountability mechanisms, Community timeframes (TRAC) method. I co-designed the TRAC method with Indigenous scholar Jeff Kanohalidoh Corntassel while we were working in partnership with a non-profit organization on a gender-based violence project across Nunangat. The TRAC method of responsive research braids Indigenous and western social scientific epistemologies at various stages of the research process and has been successfully applied in community-based research. We are further developing TRAC as a research approach to offer to scholars, practitioners, activists, and students in their future work.

Acknowledgments

The recovery of the 215 children at the Kamloops Indian Residential School in BC was publicly announced at the end of May 2021. Since then, many more children have been recovered. Indigenous communities across Canada have been experiencing tremendous grief and pain as they continue to process this horrific information. I acknowledge the ongoing impacts of residential schools and the testimonies of survivors. My thoughts and heart are with Indigenous children of the residential schools across Canada who are now making their way back home.

There are many people who have helped me intellectually, emotionally, and professionally to open my heart and mind to develop the relationships that are interconnected to the ideas written in this book. I am thankful to the First Nations Health Authority Staff in helping to arrange the interviews, and thankful to the key knowledge holders and Elders who shared knowledge that shaped the research and guided my use of the First Nations Perspective on Health and Wellness.

I am grateful to many sociologists who have worked with me, especially Bill Caroll who has greatly influenced my scholarship. I am also grateful to James Frideres for his ongoing academic support and to Doug Baer for sharing his statistical guidance. I also appreciate the suggestions on the manuscript from the Indigenous scholars invited for review, who provided engaging and thoughtful recommendations to strengthen this work. Thanks to everyone at the University for Toronto Press for their technical support: Anne Brackenbury, Susan Bindernagel, Stephanie Mazza, Robin Studniberg, and Siusan Moffat and especially Jodi Lewchuk for her tireless efforts and dedication. I am grateful for the beautiful artwork that was provided by Christi Belcourt. The work is called "The Wisdom of the Universe" and this Indigenous artwork, wrapped around the cover, reflects the main ideas presented in the book and some of the Indigenous world views also described in the book.

I am forever grateful to my family. My grandparents, parents, and children who stood by my side and offered love and encouragement. Most of all, I must thank Jeff Kanohalidoh Corntassel for holding creative space for me to dream and challenge colonial structures uninhibitedly. The Cherokee teachings of the *Sacred Fire* and *How Medicine Came to the People* and Jeff's ceremonies, songs, dances, and his notions of *Everyday Acts of Resurgence* have provided powerful ways of being in the world. Through this Cherokee knowledge sharing combined with Jeff's academic knowledge, I was able to ground my thinking and finish this work – wado and gv ge yu.

DECOLONIZING DATA

1

Introduction

The Importance of Power, Place, and Place-based Consciousness

Walking along the frozen trail from my hotel room, I could hear the crunching of the snow and feel cold air move through my nasal passages into my lungs – it was exhilarating. It was 9:30 am and still dark outside with a slight glimmer of daybreak across the frozen horizon. As I made my way to my first interview, scheduled with a shelter worker, these sounds and feelings of connection to the land helped me to remember that I had been to this place before. It had been 2001, when I was an early-career researcher working for the Government of Canada and part of a special project for Census enumeration for the Western Arctic region that brought me to Inuvik. That was my first visit, and I recall feeling a naive enthusiasm about the research process in which I was engaging. Our research had clear objectives and timelines, which I had learned were important components of a successful data collection operation. We had arranged translators in Inuvialuit to help with the face-to face interviews and garnered support letters by leadership to conduct the research in community. On the surface everything seemed fine but I distinctly remember not feeling connected with people in the community in a mutually meaningful way. Yes, we were polite and courteous in our research exchanges, but still the research process felt vacant and transactional. Something important was missing.

Twenty years later, I was walking on the same lands as a visitor and as I approached the shelter, I exchanged greetings with the shelter worker – Uvlaami. Qunuqitpit? (Hello. How are you?) We spent time exchanging about our families and I offered a gift to the shelter of children's swimming passes because I had heard that the kids loved to swim at the indoor pool but the shelter had already used up all of its supply of swim passes. This time of sharing and exchanging facilitated a deeper sense of place and community.

My point is this: while I had returned to the community to conduct research and re-apply survey methodology, the research process in itself was markedly different. I was relating differently to the participant, myself, and the process. Relationality in research is an important process that shapes the researcher, the participants, and the research process and outcomes. As the late Standing Rock Sioux scholar Vine Deloria Jr. explains, "power and place are dominant concepts – power being the living energy that inhabits and/or composes the universe, and place being the relationship of things to each other. It is much easier, in discussing Indian principles, to put these basic ideas into a simple equation: Power and place produce personality" (Deloria Jr. & Wildcat, 2001, p. 23). According to Cree scholar Gina Starblanket and Anishinaabe scholar Heidi Stark (2019), relationality is inherently fluid, dynamic, and context-dependent and tends to have multiple dimensions that include knowledge, gender, land, and modernity.

The decolonization of research methods and Indigenous resurgence in the context of individual and community health and wellness are growing, interdisciplinary fields. In this chapter, I address the questions of "How have settlers practised their relational responsibilities to decolonize Canada?" and "What are the expressions of those practices?" In doing so, I explain how research design practices need to be responsive and rooted in cultural safety practices. This means that researchers should support community-driven initiatives and work in partnership with Indigenous peoples, communities, and/or organizations in such a way as to avoid misinterpretations and misrepresentations in the knowledge inquiry process. This will support the generation of research findings that are anchored in Indigenous knowledge systems that are better equipped to inform recommendations for health, healing, and well-being. My standpoint is that the decolonization of research within social sciences requires innovative design practices that include relational allyship, partnership, honouring Indigenous ethical protocols, holding space for resurgence, and challenging power structures. These are the types of new relationships that will facilitate meaningful relationships and support Indigenous resurgence because Indigenous peoples, communities, and organizations can re-story the historical trauma on a number of levels, create new ways of understanding, and contest the deeply ingrained structures of inequality, power imbalance, and ongoing colonialism. Health initiatives for Indigenous peoples in Canada continue to reflect the values and discourse of the western medical model that are based in a needs-and-pathology paradigm that fails to provide holistic and culturally grounded solutions to Indigenous peoples.

Research into Indigenous resilience and resurgence has shown that the amount of connection to the land and community that Indigenous peoples maintain through cultural activities and "traditional" land-based activities helps them cope with the adverse impacts of colonization (Baskin, 2005; Chandler & Lalonde, 1998; Gone, 2011; Gone & Kirmayer, 2010; Kelley et al., 2012; Kirmayer et al., 2011, 2012; Kovach, 2005, 2009; Kral, 2012; Lawson-Te Aho & Liu, 2010; Million, 2013; Mundel & Chapman, 2010; Smith, 1999; Wilson & Rosenberg, 2002). However, access to and interactions with Indigenous lands, cultural activities, communities, language, and Elders, who are often the keepers of traditional knowledge, can be challenging; issues of marginalization due to systemic racism and ethnocentrism are ever-present in cities for those living a diasporic life (Peters & Anderson, 2013). Opportunities to live one's identity as an Indigenous person in an urban space can be difficult and may at times seem impossible because many Indigenous cultural practices run counter to dominant western world views (Bang et al., 2013). This chapter provides an introduction to Indigenous perspectives on well-being and social capital analysis as an analytical framework that is useful to address the conventions of state-centric processes to measure and evaluate well-being. It is argued that well-being scores are a form of structural violence on Indigenous peoples. Given that little substantive research has examined the complexities of urban Indigenous health and wellness, the chapter introduces the First Nations Perspective on Health and Wellness (FNPOW) and considers the role it has in shaping holistic health for Indigenous peoples living in urban centres across Canada. This holistic approach is important for two key reasons. First, Indigenous perspectives are often overlooked as a legitimate approach to research. As such, a holistic approach to health seeks to respect the research and personal contributions made by Indigenous scholars. Second, rather than take a deficit approach (Tuck, 2009), which often frames accounts of Indigenous health and seeks to remedy the "Indian problem" (Newhouse & McGuire-Adams, 2012), a holistic, Indigenous perspective of health considers the nature of peoples' lives (Reading & Wien, 2009). Two important questions that I address later in this book are "How is the FNPOW related to a decolonizing process and does the FNPOW generate determinants of health and wellness that advance self-determination?" and "How does understanding well-being through a decolonizing research approach support an understanding of well-being that can be of direct benefit to urban Indigenous peoples?"

Who Is Indigenous?

In Canada, the term "Aboriginal" was initially defined by the Canadian Constitution Act of 1982 (section 2[35]). In this Act, "Aboriginal peoples of Canada include the Indian, Inuit, and Métis peoples of Canada" (Canadian Constitution Act, 1982, section 2). While there is a great deal of diversity among the three main Aboriginal identity groups, the Canadian government has tended to treat each identity group homogeneously with respect to a variety of government policies and programs. Over the decades, the Census of Canada has used many different definitions to measure the construct of "Aboriginality." The most recent and widely used definition is that of "Aboriginal identity." The Aboriginal identity population in Canada includes all those who self-identify in the Census as Aboriginal and/or as registered Indians or members of an Indian Band or First Nation. The Census maintains the definition of Aboriginal people outlined in the Constitution Act and collects information accordingly; it then categorizes the Aboriginal population into fixed groups based on Census questions 18, 20, and 21 (Felligi, 1996). In the 2011 Census (Statistics Canada, 2011), question 18 asked people if they self-identify in the North American Indian, Métis, and/ or Inuit category. This question allows for multiple responses. Question 20 asked people whether they are a member of an Indian Band or First Nation and, if so, to give the name of the First Nation. Question 21 asked if a person responding to the Census is a treaty or registered Indian, which is defined as someone registered under the Indian Act. The term "Aboriginal identity" is used to include all Aboriginal identity groups: registered Indian (on- or off-reserve), Inuit, Métis, and other multiple Aboriginal non-status individuals. These categories form the basis of data, which make data on Indigenous peoples ambiguous and difficult to interpret; while much diversity exists among First Nations, Métis, and Inuit people culturally, socially, and demographically, Aboriginal people are generally marginalized within the dominant culture (Frideres, 2010).

While the word "Aboriginal" came into widespread usage in Canada after 1982, many Indigenous Nations and communities reject the term since it is defined and imposed by the state (Alfred, 2009). In fact, it is an English word defined by the government; it does not resonate with many communities and is not a word that Indigenous peoples used in the past (Alfred, 2009; Alfred & Corntassel, 2005; Smith, 2012). The word "Indigenous" encompasses a variety of approximately 370 million place-based peoples around the world and can be applied in international, transnational, or global contexts. For example, while the term "Indigenous" has become widely used, there is much diversity among Indigenous peoples. The United Nations suggests "the most fruitful approach is to identify, rather than define Indigenous peoples" (United Nations, n.d.) and for this reason the UN has not adopted an official definition of the term. In the practice of respect and in support of self-determination, this study will use the term "Indigenous" in the Canadian context to describe the "Aboriginal population" more generally except in instances when it is appropriate to use "Aboriginal" to describe a government department, organization, program, or service. In other instances, this study will also use the term "First Nation," "Métis," or "Inuit" where appropriate. Additionally, given the shortcomings of the above-mentioned terms, I recognize that referring to an Indigenous Nation's preferred community designation (especially in the language of that Nation) is the most accurate way to speak about particular Indigenous Nations.

The scholarly literature on what it means to be Indigenous focuses on identity construction and developing awareness that evaluates and deconstructs colonial contexts in present-day society in which Indigenous peoples experience and examine the wider phenomena of pan-indigenism or theories of individual self-identification. For example, Kim Anderson (2001) outlines the foundations of resistance for being Indigenous: strong families, grounding in community, connection to land, language, storytelling, and spirituality (Anderson, 2001 cited in Alfred & Corntassel, 2005). Corntassel and Bryce (2012) argue that:

> as a result of colonial encroachment into their homelands, being Indigenous today means engaging in a struggle to reclaim and regenerate one's relational, place-based existence by challenging the ongoing, destructive forces of colonization. (p. 152)

Métis scholar Chris Andersen discusses the concept of "mixedness" (Andersen, 2014) as an inherent characteristic of what it means to be a Métis person by analysing the intersection between colonialism in Métis identity and self-identification. Andersen argues that understanding what it means to be Métis is contentious and based in official processes such as the Census of Population. He argues that:

> Conflating Métis with mixedness appears logical for good reason, but as you might guess, this reason has little to do with innate coherence. Rather,

the logic is embedded in Canada's colonial histories and the relative inability of Canadian colonial administrators to think outside of their own official binaries of "white" and "Indian." (Andersen, 2014, p. 36)

These examples illustrate different ways in which scholars describe the processes by which Indigenous peoples have come to "be Indigenous," which are often situated in a colonial context. As Sayer et al. (2001) point out, being Indigenous is also an act of self-determination:

Enough cannot be said about the need for healthy communities led by healthy leaders. For any community to move ahead, healing needs to take place at various different levels including the individual, the family and at the community level. All are integrally linked with one another. (p. 23)

This is a useful interconnected way to understand Indigeneity – an understanding that is grounded in health, wellness, and how healing from colonialism needs to occur at different levels.

Indigenous Peoples and the Urban Landscape in Canada

Are there really more Indigenous peoples living in urban cities than ever before? In their report *Urbanization and Migration Patterns of Aboriginal Populations in Canada: A Half Century in Review*, Norris and Clatworthy (2011) examined three components of population growth. The first is natural increase (the difference between births and deaths); the second is net migration, (the difference between in-migrants and out-migrants); and the third is ethnic mobility (changes in ethnic identity over the life course). While the population of Indigenous peoples has been increasing in urban centres, the results of this study show that, contrary to popular opinion that claims people are leaving reserves in droves headed for the cities, the net migration rates of Indigenous peoples and First Nations in particular on reserves are positive. Positive net migration rates mean that the number of in-migrants (to reserves) exceeds the number of out-migrants and that migration cannot be the sole explanation for the growth of First Nations in metropolitan areas (Norris & Clatworthy, 2011). Rather, urban Indigenous population growth is also attributed to natural increase (the difference between fertility and mortality) and ethnic mobility whereby more people self-identify as Indigenous. As a result, "the impact of high rates of mobility due to ethnic mobility, especially among the Métis, can be significant" (Norris & Clatworthy, 2011, p. 69).

The reasons for moving away from First Nations communities differ from reasons the mainstream Canadian population moves (Aman, 2008; Clatworthy & Norris, 2007). While these findings are important, there is also a need to understand the issues surrounding mobility patterns or changes of residence within the same city or neighbourhood. This latter dimension of mobility is crucial because it constitutes an important process through which Indigenous families adjust and often readjust their housing situation in response to changes in needs and resources (Clatworthy, 2008). At a societal level, "the decision to move is the outcome of competing factors … such as education, employment and housing (availability, adequacy); institutional completeness; health facilities; and the political situation" (Clatworthy & Norris, 2007, p. 223). Factors that help draw the population to an Indigenous community include access to extended family support, education opportunities, the ability to participate in cultural activities, and a better quality of life for raising children compared to urban centres (Aman, 2008; Hull, 2006; Unicef Canada, 2009). Reserves serve as an important point of connection between urban residents in terms of maintaining a sense of connection with their family and friends, community, cultural traditions, and language (Clatworthy & Norris, 2007; Silver et al., 2006).

According to Quinless and Manmohan (2015), "almost 25 years ago, research using the 1991 Aboriginal Peoples Survey (APS) migration data found that family and housing were the key factors for moving in general" (Quinless & Manmohan, 2015, p. 115). The authors also suggest that the stage an individual is at in their life course (e.g., newlywed or owning a new home) along with other factors such as education level and gender are also associated with mobility patterns (Quinless & Manmohan, 2015). What is important to consider is that "the incidence of high mobility and its effect on Indigenous families have far-reaching social policy implications in relation to adequate program and service delivery in the areas of education, health, employment, and child care" (Quinless & Manmohan, 2015, p. 117). These factors are crucial to meeting the needs of the Indigenous diasporic community. Overall, the main drivers associated with high mobility patterns among Indigenous peoples are family, employment, housing, social services, health services, and education opportunities (Hull, 2006; Institute of Urban Studies, 2004; Norris & Clatworthy, 2003; Norris & Siggner, 2003; Quinless & Manmohan, 2015). Research studies that have been undertaken on this topic provide evidence of high geographic mobility patterns among Indigenous peoples, whether they are moving from reserves to cities or are moving frequently within neighbourhoods within the same urban centre, all of which suggest that their needs are not being addressed in terms of housing affordability, employment, education, social services, and child care. High mobility patterns are important in terms of Indigenous health and well-being and the implications of population turnover suggest "disruptive effects on individuals, families, communities, and service providers" (Quinless & Manmohan, 2015, p. 117) and further impacts on overall states of health and well-being among Indigenous peoples.

Indigenous Perspectives on the Good Life

Many Indigenous peoples understand well-being holistically, as a relational world view, through a balance of the Traditional Medicine Wheel or some rendition of it. The Traditional Medicine Wheel displays four or more dimensions of health and well-being describing the interconnectedness among physical, emotional, spiritual, and mental states of human well-being. The Medicine Wheel with its four quadrants can be linked to the environment, the community, the Nation, and even governance structures (Absolon, 2011; Kelm, 1998; Smith, 1999, 2012). The symbol of the Medicine Wheel is "an ancient symbol of the universe that reflects the cosmic order and unity of all things, variously interpreted by Aboriginal peoples from different societies" (Gray et al., 2008, p. 134). Indigenous world views of the good life are embedded in these spiritual constructs and in relationship to the earth, animal, and plant nations.

There are many words in different Indigenous languages that come to describe what Indigenous people have experienced as good living. As Frank Deer (2016) from the First Nation community Kahnawake in Quebec explains, he first heard of the term *Mino-Pimatisiwin* (which translates as the *good life* in Cree) while working in Manitoba; being of Kanien'keha:ka ancestry he wasn't familiar with the word but he was aware of the meaning. He describes Mino-Pimatisiwin (Deer & Falkenberg, 2016) as follows:

> The principal tenets associated with Mino-Pimatisiwin might be best understood not only as it applies to individual contexts but also that of communities as well. Appreciating the importance of relationships that are explored in all dimensions of Mino-Pimatisiwin gives some life to the idea that collective balance, health, harmony and growth, to name a few, is essential to the notion that what is desired is a life that is experienced in its fullest, healthiest sense. Essential to understanding how such a life might be achieved in contemporary Canadian society might be consideration to the core values of respect, sharing, and spirituality while working. (p. 2)

Newhouse and Fitzmaurice (2012) also elaborate on the good life when they explain that the Anishinaabe-Ojibwe people of the Great Lakes received knowledge, instructions, and help from the Creator that taught the importance of maintaining a balance between different aspects of their life (e.g., mental, physical, emotional, and spiritual health). This balance is an interrelationship between the inner self and the outside world with all things that when in harmony support *Mino-Bimaadiziwin* or the *good life*. This Indigenous perspective is based in an Ojibwe world view that supports a holistic approach to good health and the role of traditional medicine and spiritual healers (Simpson, 2011). Mino-Bimaadiziwin goes well beyond income and education levels, housing, and labour force activity (Newhouse & Fitzmaurice, 2012), which are how the Canadian state defines and measures well-being for Indigenous communities.

While terminology to describe good living or the good life may indeed vary across Indigenous communities by language, as Deer and Falconberg (2016) point out, the meaning is anchored in similar principles and values that are commonly understood among all Indigenous peoples. For example, the good life as outlined by Gray et al. (2008) includes many concepts such as wholeness, balance, relationships, nurturing, harmony, and healing all interconnected with respect, sharing, and spirituality (Gray et al. as cited in Deer and Falconberg, 2016). These principles are explained briefly by Gray et al. (2008, pp. 134–5) as follows:

- The concept of wholeness is about the incorporation of all aspects of life and the giving of attention and energy to each aspect within ourselves and the universe around us.
- Balance reflects the dynamic nature of relationships wherein we give attention to each aspect of the whole in a manner where one aspect is not focused on to the detriment of the other parts.
- All aspects of the whole, including the more than world, are related and these relationships require attention and nurturing; when we give energy to these relationships we nurture the connections between them. Nurturing these connections leads to health while disconnection leads to disease.
- Harmony is ultimately a process involving all entities fulfilling their obligations to each other and to themselves.
- Growth is a life-long process that involves developing aspects of oneself, such as the body, mind, heart and spirit, in a harmonious manner.

- Healing is a daily practice orientated to the restoration of wholeness, balance, relationships and harmony. It is not only focused on illness, but on disconnections, imbalances, and disharmony.

Grounded in these central ideas are the core values of the Mino-Pimatisiwin approach:

- Respect or the showing of honour, esteem, deference and courtesy to all, and not imposing our views on others
- Sharing, including the sharing of all we have to share, even knowledge and life experiences, which show that everyone is important and helps develop relationships
- Spirituality is the recognition that there is a non-physical world. It is all-encompassing in Aboriginal life and is respected in all interactions, including this helping approach, and is demonstrated through meditation, prayer, and ceremonies that guide good conduct.

The Link between Social Capital and Indigenous Well-being

There has been a plethora of research work that applies social capital analysis within Indigenous communities across Canada. This research work is dedicated to exploring the extent to which socially cohesive communities create bonds of trusting relationships that act as bridges where individuals and institutions can participate in community development projects (Chataway, 2002; Hill & Cooke, 2014; Mignone, 2003, 2009; Mignone & O'Neil, 2005b). According to Loppie-Reading and Wien (2009), the social determinants of health can be "categorized as distal (e.g., historic, political, social and economic contexts) ... intermediate (e.g., community infrastructure, resources, systems and capacities) ... and proximal (e.g., health behaviours, physical and social environment)" (p. 6). It can be argued that the good life can be seen as a form of "social capital" (Bourdieu, 1972) that reflects the network of institutions and organizations within a community to deliver programs and services and the capacity of citizens within a community to engage in the activities offered through these programs and services. Processes of capacity building eventually become larger forms of social capital derived from sites of resource at the community and individual levels and foster a sense of well-being. While there is debate in the literature about how to conceptualize and measure social capital, there is consensus about regarding it as a network of relationships between individuals and the communities in which they live that is a "resource" (Mignone, 2003; Mignone & O'Neil, 2005b) that could take a variety of forms such as good health, access to information and technological infrastructure, the practice of traditional knowledge systems, and opportunities that support social action that focuses on supporting goals at individual and community levels (Hill & Cooke, 2014). As Hill and Cooke (2014) point out:

> For some, these networks are resources held by individuals who are connected to one another and who can use these connections to access information, opportunities, or other resources. Social capital is a characteristic of the communities in which these networks and norms exist. (p. 423)

The adverse effects of contemporary colonial practices have been identified as a determinant of poor health resulting in lower states of wellness in Indigenous communities (Beavon & Jetté, 2009; Cooke, 2009; Health Canada, 2002; White, Beavon, et al., 2007; White & Maxim, 2007; White, Wingert, et al., 2007; Wingert, 2011). This has influenced Indigenous peoples' efforts to shape and determine their well-being through the regeneration of Indigenous world views as a strengths-based response to ongoing colonial practices. It is strongly recommended that traditional land-based practices through what Coulthard has termed "grounded normativity" (Coulthard, 2014) be seen as a critical component of what it means to be Indigenous. Grounded normativity conceptualizes land as a relationship to Indigenous peoples based in the obligations they have to the land. It is a reciprocal relationship involving all aspects of Indigenous life, culture, and economics (Coulthard, 2014) that, through the Indigenous resurgence movement (Alfred & Corntassel, 2005) and Indigenous research methodologies (Denzin et al., 2008), provides resistance to further dispossession and disconnection as a result of contemporary colonialism. Colonization not only impacts Indigenous relationships with land, water, and communities but also the health and well-being of Indigenous bodies themselves.

The Registered Indian Human Development Index was the first attempt by Indigenous and Northern Affairs Canada (INAC)[1] to develop systematic quantitative measures of well-being for Indigenous peoples. It is modelled after the United Nations Development

---

1 INAC will be used throughout this book, recognizing that it has now been split into two departments: Indigenous Services Canada (ISC) and Crown–Indigenous Relations and Northern Affairs Canada (CIRNAC).

Programme's Human Development Index (HDI) and Robin Armstrong's (2001) work *Geographical Patterns of Socio-Economic Well-Being of First Nations Communities in Canada* (Armstrong, 2001; Cooke, 2005). The Registered Indian Human Development Index and the work of Armstrong provided methodological guidance to the developers of the Community Well-being Index (CWB) (INAC, 2015a; O'Sullivan et al., 2007). For over a decade, the CWB has dominated the policy arena as the national wellness index used by the Government of Canada to account for levels of well-being among Indigenous and non-Indigenous communities across the country. However, the tool is severely limited in that the knowledge systems used to conceptualize well-being embedded in this framework reflect the social and cultural values of the dominant western discourse.

The values of the CWB are articulated through four main wellness dimensions: income (based on income per capita), education (based on high school and university completion rates), housing (based on housing quantity and quality), and labour force activity (based on employment and labour force participation rates) (INAC, 2015a; O'Sullivan et al., 2007). Well-being scores are calculated for Indigenous communities and the resulting numeric values assigned to each community serve to reproduce a conceptualization of well-being that represents colonial hegemonic discourse. Social capital analysis is also a useful analytical framework to understanding the good life when we consider that in a Bourdieusian sense, well-being scores exert a form of structural violence on Indigenous peoples because the scores exercise colonial power over Indigenous peoples by legitimizing western ways of thinking about well-being over Indigenous ways of "being well." The system produces an index score that represents and explicitly defines what well-being is and how it should be conceptualized for Indigenous peoples, thus failing to integrate Indigenous knowledge systems about health and wellness. This knowledge has been internalized by many Indigenous communities and peoples, which further colonizes their inner life-worlds (Browne et al., 2005) and serves to validate thinking about *what does* and *what does not* constitute Indigenous wellness.

Current threats to language practices and traditional activities (e.g., hunting, trapping, and harvesting for Indigenous peoples) are threats to maintaining a strong sense of cultural identity while also negatively impacting states of well-being at both the individual and community levels for urban Indigenous peoples (Blackstock, 2009; Hallett et al., 2007; Ledogar & Fleming 2008a; Norris, 2006; O'Sullivan, 2010). Despite its continued usage, it is obvious that the CWB is limited in its ability to account for Indigenous well-being. Many scholars have critiqued the CWB and the model it was conceptualized from, which is the Human Development Index, for being narrowly focused, redundant, and limited in how and what it measures by way of indicators of Indigenous wellness (Gracey & King, 2009; Kirmayer et al., 2003; McGillivray, 1991; Wilson, 2008). In fact, the First Nations Health Authority (FNHA) and the First Nations Information Governance Centre (FNIGC) have already discontinued the use of this tool (FNIGC, 2012), recognizing that tracking and measuring changes to well-being over time for Indigenous communities need to be from an Indigenous standpoint. Otherwise, what do we *really* know about the factors that shape the social determinants of health and wellness for Indigenous peoples? This question is important but has not been adequately addressed in the literature on the social determinants of Indigenous health and wellness.

The First Nations Perspective on Health and Wellness (FNPOW) is a perspective that can be applied by researchers and was developed by the FNHA in direct consultation with First Nations communities in British Columbia, providing a lens by which to explore the effects of various social determinants on the well-being of Indigenous peoples residing in the urban landscape across Canada. The FNHA was created as an act of self-determination based on what Indigenous scholars have referred to as an ongoing resistance struggle based in anger and resentment of a colonial relationship that has characterized Indigenous–settler relations (Coulthard, 2014; Denis, 2015). In 2005, BC First Nations political leadership signed the Leadership Accord, which was a formal agreement of a working relationship among the three main First Nations political organizations in BC (the BC Assembly of First Nations, First Nations Summit, and Union of BC Indian Chiefs) and is now referred to as the First Nations Leadership Council (FNHA, 2016a). In 2013, the FNHA was created out of the determination to address long-standing health disparities for First Nations in British Columbia and close the health gap. A tripartite agreement between the Province of British Columbia, the Government of Canada, and BC First Nations recognizes that the FNHA is "the province-wide health authority in British Columbia that assumes all responsibility for programs, services and budgetary considerations for the health and well-being of BC's First Nations and Indigenous peoples" (FNHA, n.d., p. 8). The mandate of the FNHA focuses on health promotion and disease prevention and the organization. The FNHA is "working to reform the way health care is delivered to BC First Nations … based in political representation and advocacy through the First Nations Health Council and the First Nations Health Directors Association" (FNHA, n.d., p. 8).

2

The Impacts of Colonization on Indigenous Health and Well-being

I want to get rid of the Indian problem. Our objective is to continue until there is not a single Indian in Canada that has not been absorbed into the body politic, and there is no Indian question, and no Indian Department. That is the whole object of this Bill.

– Duncan Campbell Scott, 1920[1]

What followed from the above-referenced statement was a period in Indigenous–settler relations of forced relocation, oppression, and settlement on the state-designed reservation system. Reserves, residential schools, the Indian Act, and the creation of the Department of Indian Affairs are not just shadow moments that darken Canadian history; these are shameful testaments to the inhumane treatment of Indigenous peoples by the Canadian government. The ongoing processes of colonization continue with the infringement of Indigenous land rights and the legacy of the residential school system (Bastien, 2004; Bastien et al., 2003; Daschuk, 2013; Milloy, 1999) that continues through "transgenerational effects of historical trauma," (Gone et al., 2014, p. 301) or transgenerational trauma.

There has been an ongoing history of state violence and harm against Indigenous peoples and, despite the 2015–19 Liberal government's efforts to advance a reconciliation agenda, Indigenous peoples still experience social, economic, political, and health inequalities. This chapter describes Government of Canada assimilation policy, the reserve system, and residential schools and provides a critical review

---

1 Duncan Campbell Scott was the superintendent of Department of Indian Affairs from 1913–1932 and is known today for assimilating First Nations peoples.

of the impacts of colonization on Indigenous peoples' health in Canada. The impacts on Indigenous peoples have and continue to be many, with the loss of culture (outlawing the practice of traditional ceremonies), loss of land, and loss of children (residential schools and children in state care). This legacy of residential schools and assimilation policies is expressed by transgenerational trauma that continues to be passed down between generations through processes of cultural transmission (Castellano & Archibald, 2007). This had and continues to have significant adverse impacts on Indigenous peoples that are evident in dispossession from the land, language, and culture and in the manifestation of health disparities situating Indigenous peoples in a subaltern position. The aim of this chapter is to present a historical narrative and theoretical framework from which to understand contemporary Indigenous health conditions and wellness. A central theme of this chapter is the ongoing processes of colonialism through the legacies of the residential school system, Indian Act, Department of Indian Affairs, and ongoing state-centric colonial practices, which all have negative impacts on different states of Indigenous well-being.

Settler-state Policy and Indigenous Peoples

There is growing recognition that Canadian public policy should promote Indigenous well-being as opposed to merely addressing social problems through the lens of a needs assessment approach to improving the lives of Indigenous peoples (Beavon & Jetté, 2009; Cooke, 2009; White & Maxim, 2007; White, Wingert, et al., 2007; Wingert, 2011). This means going beyond identifying the problems and challenges in Indigenous communities in terms of "gaps" to a focus on emphasizing community capacity initiatives. It means suspending damaged-centred research that emphasizes peoples' pain and frames the community as depleted (Tuck, 2009). The Liberal government of Canada (2015) publicly announced several commitments to advancing the welfare of Indigenous peoples. The most important of these is reflected in several recent actions aimed at enhancing Indigenous individual and community well-being through the Truth and Reconciliation Commission's ninety-four Calls to Action (Truth and Reconciliation Commission [TRC], 2015). In February 2014, the Government of Canada and the National Association of Friendship Centres reached a new funding agreement through the new Urban Aboriginal Strategy. This agreement places an emphasis on increasing well-being and economic engagement by affording the National Association of Friendship Centres access to new resources in terms of policy areas and the pursuit of new relationships. Specifically, the Urban Aboriginal Strategy is a strategic framework implemented by the former Department of Indigenous and Northern Affairs Canada, now called the Department of Indigenous Services Canada, to address urban Indigenous issues in the multijurisdictional environment with multiple stakeholders throughout Canada's urban centres. The strategy is a manifestation of previous efforts outlined in the Economic Action Plan 2012 that focused on increasing urban Aboriginal participation in the economy (Flaherty, 2012) by funding and facilitating activities that lead to greater collaboration between partners through two major programs: Community Capacity Support and Urban Partnerships. The programming is comprised of two funding streams: $23 million for Community Capacity Support and $20 million for Urban Partnerships annually (National Association of Friendship Centres, 2016).

There is a wide range of contemporary concerns over the relation between settler-state and Indigenous relations in Canada, particularly with regard to ongoing colonial practices to address Indigenous health and wellness in Canada. Critical reflection on research methodologies has something important to add to these issues and offers applied methods that centre Indigenous knowledge systems to address health inequalities. First Nations' relationships with the Canadian government, which are characterized by colonial forms of governance, have influenced their health and resulted in widespread epidemics of infectious diseases, the denigration of Indigenous governing systems, dispossession from the land, dispossession from culture and identity, degradation of health care, and violence against women and children (Aboriginal Affairs Working Group, 2010; Bryce, 1907; Daschuk, 2013; Hutchinson, 2006; Kelm, 1998; Milloy, 1999; Mosby, 2013). The federal government in Canada has not addressed the issues of overcrowded and inadequate housing, poor water quality, and unsanitary living conditions that have resulted in the continued spread of disease, pathology, and poor health among Indigenous peoples (Daschuk, 2013; Kelm, 1998; Lavoie et al., 2008; Mosby, 2013). There are many reasons why the federal government has not adequately addressed these concerns. While it has been touted that Canada is in an era of reconciliation, the truth of the matter is that many Indigenous peoples continue to experience ongoing colonial oppression that contributes to severe health inequalities.

Assimilation Policy and Poor Health Outcomes

The Royal Proclamation of 1763 recognized Indian Nations as self-governing entities but there was a shift of imperial policy from 1830 to 1850 that resulted in Canada's assimilationist Indian policy (Milloy,

1999). In 1857, the Act for the Gradual Civilization of Indians was passed and the government's new Indian policy of assimilation was set to control Indian Nations. In 1867, the British North America Act, section 91(24) gave the federal government legislative jurisdiction, authoritative power, and fiduciary responsibility for the Indian Nations (Milloy, 1999). In 1876, the Indian Act consolidated pre-Confederation legislation into a nation-wide framework that gave the Department of Indian Affairs legal jurisdiction for administrative power to rule over Indigenous peoples and lands and provided legislative structures that were used to develop a colonial system to subordinate Indigenous peoples (Kelm, 1998; Miller, 1991; Milloy, 1999). Under colonial rule Indigenous peoples became wards of the state and, as Fleras and Elliott (1996) point out, through various positive and negative sanctions, "Indian Affairs sought to destroy the cultural basis of aboriginal society; transform aboriginal people through exposure to Christianity and arts of civilization; assimilate them into society as self-reliant and productive citizens" (Fleras & Elliott, 1996, p. 203). The Department of Indians Affairs was the central branch for the administration of Indigenous peoples; the Indian Act and British North America Act (Canada's constitution) worked to segregate Indigenous and non-Indigenous peoples. The impacts of colonization through this colonial network system resulted in institutionalized violence that attempted to disrupt and destroy Indigenous relationships to land, family, community, and cultural practices through the residential school system, reserves, and systemic racism. This institutionalized violence against Indigenous families and Nations perpetuated the view that Indigenous peoples were inferior to non-Indigenous peoples (Kelm, 1998; Miller, 1991; Milloy, 1999).

The Indian Reserve System

The Department of Indian Affairs set up a system of reservations and settlements that was intended to control and segregate Indigenous peoples (Harris, 2003). Communities were forced to relocate to remote locations with severe climate conditions. Indigenous peoples experienced isolation and widespread disease, and even today many reserves in Canada are in a continued state of crisis with insufficient waste disposal, unsafe drinking water, and low levels of food security (Daschuk, 2013). Daschuk (2013) states:

> Half-hearted relief measures during the famine of 1878–80 and after, which kept plains people in a constant state of hunger, not only undermined the government's half-baked self-sufficiency initiative but also illustrated the

moral and legal failures of the crown's treaty commitment to provide assistance in the case of a widespread famine on the plains. (p. 101)

Daschuk's (2013) work clearly shows that over the past century public health researchers have been aware that reserves exist in harsh environments and unsafe conditions, all of which continue to contribute to high rates of disease, starvation, suicide, alcoholism, and other forms of trauma but this awareness was dismissed as "officials began to interpret the chronic bad health of the Indigenous population as a condition of their race" (Daschuk, 2013, p. 185). The legacy of colonialism is observed in the negative effects of a colonial government that has perpetuated communities' economic, social, and political dependency on the state (Alfred, 2009). The reserve and settlement system is an institutionalized form of segregation with long-term effects and "while Canadians see themselves as world leaders in social welfare, health care, and economic development ... even basics such as clean drinking water remain elusive for some [Indigenous] communities" (Daschuk, 2013, p. 186).

While the impact of colonization manifests differently among the distinct Indigenous groups in Canada, similar historical and contemporary social determinants have shaped the health and well-being of individuals, families, communities, and Nations. For example, the impact of colonialism is similar among all Indigenous peoples who experienced policies such as the Indian Act and residential schools but "in particular to First Nations communities in Canada, social cohesion faced a major decline during the period of residential schooling and in the longer term due to colonialism" (Reading et al., 2007, p. 21) and this has been detrimental to the health and well-being of First Nations people. According to the TRC, "Reconciliation as an ongoing process of establishing and maintaining respectful relationships and a critical part of this process involves repairing damaged trust by making apologies, providing reparations, and following through with concrete actions that demonstrate real change" (TRC, 2015, p. 16). These changes must respect the right to self-determination.

The Residential School System

There were 139 recognized residential schools in Canada (see figure 1). Gordon Residential School, the last federally run facility, closed in 1996.

It is estimated that 150,000 children were taken from their families and forced to attend residential school (TRC, 2015) and approximately 6,000 children died – but according to Truth and Reconciliation

Figure 1. Distribution of residential schools in Canada

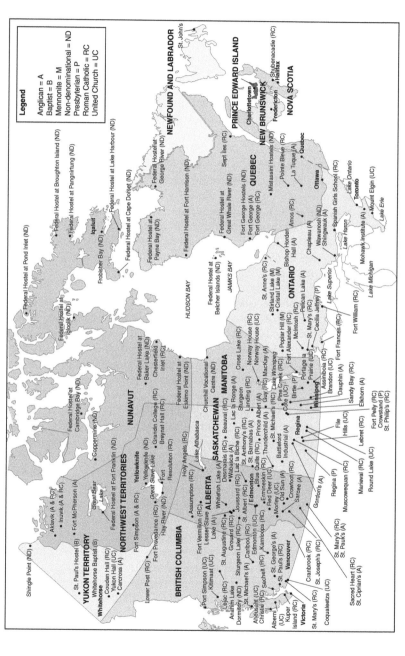

Data from INAC, 2016

Commissioner Murray Sinclair, the federal government stopped count-
ing in the 1920s (Puxley, 2015). The purpose of the residential school
system was to eliminate all aspects of Indigenous culture and abol-
ish Indigenous values, beliefs, cultures, traditions, and land through
church-run schools (Daschuk, 2013). This was a calculated strategy by
which the Government of Canada attempted to assimilate Indigenous
children into the dominant culture (Miller, 1991; Milloy, 1999). The residential school system was the main approach of the Government of
Canada's Aboriginal policy:

> When Canada was created as a country in 1867, churches were already
> operating a small number of boarding schools for Indigenous peoples.
> As settlement moved westward in the 1870s, Roman Catholic and Prote-
> stant missionaries established missions and small boarding schools across
> the Prairies, in the North, and in British Columbia. ... In 1883, the federal
> government established three large residential schools for First Nation
> children in western Canada. In the following years, the system grew dra-
> matically. (TRC, 2015, p. 3)

Students wore uniforms and followed regimented timetables, ties to
family were cut, and physical and sexual abuse were common (Blackstock et al., 2004; Milloy, 1999; Morrisette, 1994; Rogers et al., 2012). The
residential school system was based on an assumption that European
civilization and Christianity were superior to Indigenous peoples and
their culture (Kelm, 1998; Miller, 1991; Milloy, 1999). The schools were
strict and Indigenous children were regarded as savage and prohibited
from speaking their native languages. The 2015 TRC reports that the
missionaries who ran the schools played prominent roles in the church-
led campaigns to ban Aboriginal spiritual practices, for example, the
Potlatch and the Sun Dance (TRC, 2015). Abuse at many of the schools
was widespread; emotional and psychological abuse were constant,
physical abuse was used as a form of punishment on a regular basis,
and sexual abuse occurred quite often and this "abusive punishment
often prompted children to run away" (TRC, 2015, p. 103). According
to the TRC (2015), survivors recall being beaten and strapped and other
severe physical assaults such as whipping and second-degree burns and
other severe punishments for speaking their native languages. These
abuses, along with inadequate food and health care, resulted in high
death rates among Indigenous children (TRC, 2015).

   In 1907, government medical inspector P.H. Bryce released his con-
troversial *Report on the Indian Schools of Manitoba and the North-West
Territories* reporting that 24 per cent of previously healthy Aboriginal

children across Canada were dying in residential schools of tuberculosis (Bryce, 1907). Bryce believed that the state needed to address this high death rate (Bryce, 1907). This figure did not include children who died at home, where they were frequently sent when critically ill. Bryce reported that anywhere from 47 per cent (on the Peigan Reserve in Alberta) to 75 per cent (from File Hills Boarding School in Saskatchewan) of the students discharged from residential schools died shortly after returning home (Bryce, 1907, 1922). Bryce was "forcibly" retired from the civil service in 1921, at which point he revealed to Canadians the treatment of Indigenous peoples by the Government of Canada. In 1922, he published a critical review of the management of Aboriginal policy and Indigenous affairs in Canada entitled *The Story of a National Crime*, which was a document that outlined systematic attempts by the Department of Indian Affairs to hide health information of Indigenous peoples from the general public. Bryce (1922) argued that Duncan Campbell Scott, the deputy superintendent of the department of Indian affairs, in particular had consistently failed to acknowledge and address the health needs of Indigenous peoples when he states that as a result of "Mr. D.C. Scott and his advice to the then Deputy Minister, no action was taken by the Department to give effect to the recommendations made" (p. 5).

Indigenous peoples have experienced what has been described as "cultural genocide" (Truth Commission into Genocide in Canada, 2001, p. 12). Experiments were run on Indigenous children in residential schools that negatively impacted their health and well-being (Mosby, 2013). For example, Ian Mosby (2013) describes government-sponsored biomedical and nutritional experimentation on Indigenous children at six Canadian residential schools, as well as in Northern Manitoban Indigenous communities. The research revealed details about government experiments conducted on at least 1,300 Aboriginal people – most of them children – who were used as test subjects in the 1940s and 1950s by researchers probing the effectiveness of vitamin supplements (Mosby, 2013). This resulted in a lost generation who survived the residential school system, which severely altered social organization and family structures and overall states of well-being at both the individual and community levels (Truth Commission into Genocide in Canada, 2001). Residential schools had a devastating impact on Indigenous knowledge systems based in traditional customs and practices.

As another example, in his book *Clearing the Plains: Disease, Politics of Starvation and the Loss of Aboriginal Life*, James Daschuk (2013) describes that, after 1869, starvation and the spread of disease were used deliberately to make room for non-Indigenous settlement on the northern plains. Daschuk identifies the roots of the current health disparity between the Indigenous and mainstream populations in western Canada and explains that this gap in health outcomes has historical roots in the policies and practices of Canada towards Indigenous peoples. As Daschuk (2013) explains, years of hunger coincided with extermination of the bison and relocation of groups to reserves, creating ecological conditions that laid the foundation for rampant disease with no food aid from the government (Daschuk, 2013). The loss of traditional Indigenous food sources and the introduction of European diseases are linked to numerous socio-economic historical and cultural circumstances. Daschuk (2013) outlines the transmission patterns of smallpox, trade networks in the preparation and sale of furs, and the introduction of new technologies (e.g., horses, steamboats, and the Canadian Pacific Railway) all as factors that he points out contributed to the introduction and spread of disease.

Cultural genocide is commonly understood as the destruction of those structures and practices that allow the group to continue as a group. According to the TRC (2015), "when a State engages in cultural genocide the administration sets out to destroy the socio-political institutions of the targeted group, land is seized, and populations are forcibly transferred and their movement is restricted" (p. 1). Cultural traditions are denied, speaking Indigenous languages is not allowed and "families are disrupted to prevent the transmission of cultural values and identity from one generation to the next" (TRC, 2015, p. 1). In effect, the TRC officially recognizes that the Government of Canada destroyed the culture of many Indigenous communities (TRC, 2015). The legacy of colonialism continues to shape states of well-being at individual and community levels for Indigenous peoples. The residential school system is now symbolic of ongoing colonization and a socio-historical event with a legacy that reintroduces past trauma into Indigenous communities through what has been called "intergenerational trauma" (TRC, 2015).

Historical Trauma for Generations to Come

Upon signing the United Nations Universal Declaration of Human Rights in December 1948, Canada's government was forced to re-examine its treatment of Indigenous peoples for the first time (Hawthorn, 1967). In 1951, the Indian Act was changed so that most laws banning main cultural traditions such as Potlatches and pow-wows were removed. By the 1960s, it was well documented that, compared to non-Indigenous peoples in Canada, Indigenous peoples were facing greater rates of poverty, higher infant mortality rates, lower life expectancy rates, and lower levels of income and education (White, Wingert, et al., 2007). In 1967, Hawthorn's report *A Survey of the Contemporary Indians of Canada: Economic, Political, Educational Needs and Policies* found that Indigenous peoples were the most disadvantaged and marginalized population in Canadian society, which Hawthorn attributed to years of failed government policy and the residential school system (Hawthorn, 1967). This led during the period of 1969–1970 to what are commonly known as the White and Red Papers. The White Paper (officially referred to as Statement of the Government of Canada on Indian Policy) was issued shortly after Prime Minister Pierre Trudeau was elected in 1968 (Weaver, 1993). The Trudeau government issued a White Paper on Aboriginal policy that argued that Canada should not negotiate treaties with Indigenous peoples because it was Trudeau's position that treaties were only signed between sovereign nations (Weaver, 1993). The Trudeau government did not agree with Indigenous land rights claims based on the notion that they were too broad and unspecific (Weaver, 1993). In 1970, the Alberta Indian Association and the National Indian Brotherhood responded with their own document named *Citizens Plus* and otherwise known as the Red Paper (Cardinal, 1999; Weaver, 1993). The Hawthorn report "failed to emphasize Indian participation in the policy making process" (Weaver, 1993, p. 89) and the Red Paper countered all of the proposals of the White Paper but expressed the need to recognize Aboriginal title and treaty rights (Weaver, 1993). In 1973, the Supreme Court's decision on the Calder case forced the government to radically change its policies and positions (Cardinal, 1999; Weaver, 1993).[2] This case is important and points to fact that today Indigenous lands in British Columbia are unceded.

Acts of Reconciliation

The 1996 Royal Commission on Aboriginal Peoples

In the summer of 1990 the Mohawks of Kanesatake, the Government of Quebec, the Quebec provincial police, and the Canadian military entered a violent confrontation over the Town of Oka's plan to develop

2 In 1967, Frank Calder sued the provincial Government of British Columbia, declaring that Nisga'a title to their lands had never been lawfully extinguished through treaty. The Supreme Court's 1973 decision was the first time that the Canadian legal system acknowledged the existence of Aboriginal title to land outside of colonial law (Cardinal, 1999).

a golf course on Mohawk burial grounds located in a forested area known as "The Pines" that is considered traditional territory of the Mohawk peoples (Alfred, 1995). What started as a peaceful act of resistance by Mohawk land protectors erupted into violence and the "Oka Crisis," as this historical event is commonly referred to, resulted in a seventy-eight-day standoff. Cox and Nilsen (2014) refer to this event as militant particularism, which is:

> those forms of struggle that can emerge if such a process of extraction and development takes place: when local rationalities are transformed from tacit potentialities to explicitly oppositional practices deployed in conflictual encounters with dominant groups. (p. 76)

This form of militant particularism completely shifted national and international thinking about Indigenous–settler relations in Canada (Alfred, 1995). Certainly, the outcomes of the Oka Crisis have been many but one in particular was that the Government of Canada created a Royal Commission to further examine the state of affairs of Indigenous peoples in Canada as a way to better understand the relationship dynamics. In 1996, the Royal Commission on Aboriginal Peoples (RCAP) put forward a vision of reconciliation that clearly outlined a number of recommendations to support the relationship between Aboriginal peoples and the Crown. The report concluded that the policy of assimilation was a failure and that Canada must look to the historical treaty relationship to establish a new relationship between Aboriginal and non-Aboriginal peoples "accompanied by a rebalancing of power" (RCAP, 1996b, p. 1).

The Royal Commission on Aboriginal Peoples (RCAP, 1996a) emphasized that Aboriginal peoples' right to self-determination is essential to upholding Canada's constitutional obligations to Aboriginal peoples and compliance with international human rights law. The report described reconciliation as a relationship between the Government of Canada and Indigenous peoples in such a way that two main things needed to happen. "First, there has to be a sincere acknowledgment by non-Aboriginal people of the injustices of the past … second there must be a profound and unambiguous commitment to establishing a new relationship for the future" (RCAP, 1996b, p. 3). Although the commission released a five-volume comprehensive report detailing the reasons for the how and why of reconciliation, there have been ongoing challenges in developing a national framework of reconciliation. While Indigenous peoples, governments, and the courts agree that reconciliation is needed, "it has been difficult to create the conditions for reconciliation to flourish" (TRC, 2015, p. 186). In 1996, the *Report of the Royal Commission on Aboriginal Peoples* initiated a national process of reconciliation but the vast majority of the recommendations from the 1996 Royal Commissions on Aboriginal peoples were never implemented by the Canadian government (TRC, 2015). "In 2015, as the Truth and Reconciliation Commission of Canada wrapped up its work, the country now has a rare second chance to seize a lost opportunity for reconciliation" (TRC, 2015, p. 7).

The 2015 Truth and Reconciliation Commission

In 2008, the Harper government apologized to Indigenous peoples affected by the residential school system and recognized the ongoing negative impacts of residential schools on Indigenous communities. The TRC was created following Prime Minister Stephan Harper's apology to compensate for harms and to educate Canadians about what happened in the residential school system. The Commission was also created to investigate the impacts of the schools on Indigenous peoples in Canada through truth-telling forums for attendees of residential schools, which occurred at various locations throughout Canada (TRC, 2015). In July 2015, *Honouring the Truth, Reconciling for the Future*, the final report of the TRC, was published. The 2015 TRC was established through the 2007 Indian Residential Schools Settlement Agreement to engage in a dialogue process with Indigenous peoples across Canada and to listen to the testimonies from Indigenous peoples who attended residential schools. In all, the TRC issued ninety-four Calls to Action to the Government of Canada (TRC, 2015).

The 2015 TRC's mandate focused on truth through story to open the conversation about the reconciliation component of the report (TRC, 2015). The report recognizes that the residential school system has had on ongoing effect on Indigenous peoples and that reconciliation is not just an Indigenous problem but is a problem of national importance (TRC, 2015). After I attended TRC-related events in Ottawa during 2015 and also read the ninety-four Calls to Action, my own interpretations of the report focused on two questions: "How does trauma determine the health and wellness outcomes of urban Indigenous peoples?" and "How do decolonizing methodologies produce determinants of health and wellness that support self-determination?"

To some people, reconciliation is the re-establishment of a relationship; however, a conciliatory relationship has never existed between the First Peoples of Turtle Island and the Government of Canada (Corntassel et al, 2009; Coulthard, 2014; Simpson 2011). To others, reconciliation as outlined in the 2015 TRC report is understood in the context of government assimilation policy, the Department of Indian Affairs, the reserve system, and the residential school system. According to the 2015 TRC report, reconciliation is about establishing and "maintaining a mutually respectful relationship between Aboriginal and non-Aboriginal peoples ... in order for that to happen, there has to be awareness of the past, acknowledgment of the harm that has been inflicted, and action to change behaviour" (TRC, 2015, p. 7).

Through colonization, traditional teachings and culture came under attack from members of the dominant culture. For example, after the signing of treaties in the late nineteenth century, the residential school system was established by religious missionaries under the direction of the Canadian government (TRC, 2015). Indian residential schools, which operated from 1763 to 1996, were intended to remove Indigenous children from their families and communities to assimilate, civilize, and Christianize the students (TRC, 2015). This system of domination resulted in many atrocities and a nearly complete cultural genocide that robbed Indigenous children of their language, traditional ways of knowing, identity, and self-worth, severing relationships with their families and their connectedness to the land (Blackstock, 2012).

In her book *Life Beside Itself: Imagining Care in the Canadian Arctic*, Lisa Stevenson (2014) provides an anthropological narrative that outlines two historical moments of the impacts of Canadian policies and biopolitical forms: care of the Inuit during the tuberculosis epidemic (1940s–early 1960s) and the suicide epidemic (1980s–present). It explores care in a way that embraces the possibility of being multiple things at the same time. It opens up a conversation to living and thinking about images differently in the way we relate with each other and questions what it really means to be alive in the context of different forms of care. Stevenson (2014) explains that when we relate differently to each other "there is something to be learned by juxtaposing the response of the Canadian State to the Tuberculosis epidemic – which is often couched in humanitarian or life-saving terms" (p. 22).

With the 2015 TRC Calls to Action as well as Canada's endorsement of the United Nations Declaration on the Rights of Indigenous Peoples (UNDRIP) (2007), many people have come to understand that we are living in an era of reconciliation. Amid this backdrop, detailed and culturally relevant analysis of the determinants of Indigenous health and well-being is important in understanding conversations around reconciliation but also everyday acts of Indigenous resurgence (Corntassel, 2012; Hunt & Holmes, 2015; Reading et al., 2007; Regan, 2010). Cindy

Blackstock, Gitxsan child advocate and Indigenous scholar, argues that "reconciliation means not saying sorry twice" (Blackstock, 2012, p. 1). Paulette Regan, the director of research for the TRC, takes this one step further in *Unsettling the Settler Within, Indian Residential Schools* by reminding us that Indigenous settler relations in Canada have been built on "violence, abuse and racism that is a fundamental denial of the human dignity and rights of Indigenous peoples" (Regan, 2010, p. 5). Therefore, truth and reconciliation can only occur when settlers acknowledge and take responsibility for the legacy of systemic violence that is at the core of the residential school system (Regan, 2010). All of this suggests that reconciliation conversations are incomplete without understanding the colonial past and without understanding Indigenous world views, which are based in practices of collectivism, non-ownership, living in balance and harmony with nature, and an overall perspective that sees everything as interconnected (Reading et al., 2007; Regan, 2010).

If Canada were ranked truly on well-being based on First Nations health and well-being, quantitative measures like the Human Development Index (HDI) and CWB would not mask the deeper harms that are being caused. In fact, when we measure the progress of the ninety-four Calls to Action of the TRC by "Beyond 94" (published in March 19, 2018 and updated periodically by the Canadian Broadcasting Corporation [CBC, n.d.]), we clearly observe that as of April 2021 only ten of ninety-four Calls to Action had been completed. Of these ten Calls to Action, none are related to child welfare, education, health, or justice but rather focus on sports, media, and language. Indeed, a careful review of this document shows that overall there is a general lack of progress. The status of many Calls to Action is either "Not Started" or "In Progress," which will have continued negative impacts on health and well-being:

> Most of the funds committed – $1.08 billion – are earmarked for 2019 and beyond, after the next federal election, when a new government might have different priorities. The commitment came in response to a February 2018 non-compliance order in which the Canadian Human Rights Tribunal found the federal government was not adequately funding the agencies. (CBC, n.d.)

Palmater (as cited in Antony et al., 2017) provides startling statistics to illustrate the extent of chronic underfunding of essential social services, lack of basic infrastructure, and the discrimination experienced in health and justice services by Indigenous peoples. Palmater (as cited in Antony et al., 2017) integrates various sources to delineate a national statistical portrait and explains that:

> More than 113 First Nations are without clean drinking water; forty-eight percent of all children in foster care are First Nations; sixty percent of First Nations children live in poverty. In the last decade there has been a 90 percent increase in the rate of imprisonment of Indigenous women in Canada; if nothing changes in terms of schooling resources, it will take 28 years to close the education gap between First Nations and Canadians; if nothing changes, it will take 63 years to close the income gap between First Nations and Canadians. (p. 51)

The historical harms on Indigenous peoples, communities, and lands are well documented. For example, in their book *Accounting for Geno-cide: Canada's Bureaucratic Assault on Aboriginal People*, Neu and Therrien (2003) explain that "relationships between Indigenous peoples and governments are filtered and managed through a complex field of bureaucratized manipulations, controlled by soft technologies such as strategic planning, law and accounting" (p. 5). The consequences of racist policies, government misrepresentations, and reckless corporations continue to disregard the rights of Indigenous peoples and use the legal system to force Indigenous peoples into a position of scarcity, dependency on state welfare, social crisis, and cycles of poverty. Colonial practices, especially in terms of policies and attitudes, have colonized Indigenous peoples' bodies and this chapter provided a contextual understanding of how Indigenous peoples' experiences with colonialism have impacted their overall states of health and wellness. Indigenous self-determination and resurgence are essential steps along the pathway to freedom.

3

Decolonizing Bodies and a Self-governing Health System

The aim of this chapter is to present a historical narrative and theoretical framework from which to understand contemporary Indigenous health conditions and wellness using a critical theory approach to health and wellness coupled with a holistic understanding of health and wellness that relies on the FNPOW. The FNPOW supports the interrelationship and balance among physical, mental, emotional, and spiritual aspects and "Aboriginal community development requires that Aboriginal people first heal, which requires, among other things, that they go through a process of decolonization" (Silver et al., 2006, p. 2). This chapter provides a contextual understanding of how Indigenous peoples' experiences with colonialism have impacted their overall states of health and wellness. Given that little substantive research has examined the complexities of urban Indigenous health and wellness, this chapter makes an important contribution to the urban Indigenous health literature by examining the role that the FNPOW plays in shaping holistic health. This holistic approach is important for two key reasons. First, Indigenous perspectives and knowledges are often overlooked in terms of their important research contributions. As such, a holistic approach to health seeks to respect the research and personal contributions made by Indigenous scholars and activists. Second, rather than take a deficit approach, which often frames negative accounts of Indigenous health as an articulation of the "Indian problem" (Newhouse & McGuire-Adams, 2012), a holistic, Indigenous perspective of health considers the everyday nature of peoples' lives (Loppie-Reading & Wien, 2009).

The Canadian government is committed to enhancing Indigenous well-being as a way to build investments in the Canadian economy; current conceptual frameworks and measurement tools such as the CWB used to track and measure changes in community well-being do not reflect Indigenous ways of knowing and well-being, which are based on a holistic view that balances the physical, mental, emotional, and spiritual dimensions of wellness (Blackstock, 2009; Denis, 2015; Ledogar & Fleming, 2008b, 2008c; McGillivray, 1991). The fact that Indigenous peoples are experiencing a health crisis is well-supported in the literature (Absolon, 2011; Ahenakew, 2011, 2012; Blackstock, 2009; Castellano, 2006; Frideres & Gadacz, 2006; Kirmayer et al., 2011). As Ahenakew (2011, 2012) points out, while many Indigenous peoples have stated they have been excessively researched, social research has in many ways contributed to the pathologization of Indigenous states of well-being (Ahenakew, 2011, 2012) and the post-colonization of Indigenous peoples has contributed to a general mistrust of western researchers (Absolon, 2011; Linklater, 2014; Smith, 1999, 2012).

Indigenous Well-being and Urban Life

More Indigenous peoples in Canada now live in urban centres than on reserves, an urbanization trend that is most pronounced in western Canadian cities such as Winnipeg, Edmonton, and Vancouver (Peters et al., 2013; Quinless, 2009). It has been estimated that over half (57%) of the Indigenous population in Canada currently resides in urban centres and population estimates project continued growth in the coming years (Statistics Canada, 2012). Understanding urban well-being for Indigenous peoples is important when we consider that recent figures also show that most urban Indigenous peoples live far below the low-income cut-off and experience higher rates of unemployment, poor school attendance among youth, high rates of drug and alcohol abuse, teen pregnancy, violence, prostitution, and a number of other socio-economic and cultural issues that impact overall states of personal and community wellness (Environics Institute, 2010; Guimond et al., 2012; Statistics Canada, 2012). The concept of well-being appears to be a central component of new strategies related to Indigenous engagement in the Canadian economy with the intention of stimulating long-term, sustainable economic development. However, one emerging issue that is overlooked in policy discussions and recent government strategies is that "well-being" is a complex and elusive concept with several interrelated subjective and objective dimensions. This makes it difficult to define the concept precisely. This becomes clear when we consider that what constitutes "well-being can mean different things to different people at different times" (Quinless, 2014, p. 21) or that how well-being is conceptualized and the measures used to define and implement well-being are relative and have been inconsistent over time (Quinless, 2015).

Current research trends indicate a shift in how the concept of Indigenous well-being is conceptualized (Chretien, 2010) in terms of the dimensions and indicators used to define and measure it. Several subjective and objective aspects of well-being operate on different levels, including individual, family, community, and even national levels (Quinless, 2015). These are further comprised of a variety of complex and interrelated factors, such as early education, employment, food security, social cohesion, social inclusion, access to health services and programs, housing conditions, various forms of income support, the physical environment, occupation and working conditions, personal health practices, parenting and life skills, and gender (Cooke et al., 2008; Hill & Cooke, 2014; Quinless, 2015; White, Beavon, et al., 2007; White, Wingert, et al., 2007; White et al., 2009). It is well documented in the literature that well-being includes socio-economic indicators such as education and income but has been also extended to include numerous socio-cultural factors that influence an individual throughout their life course. Socio-cultural activities could include, for example, participation in cultural activities such as arts and crafts, sacred healing ceremonies, land-based traditions of hunting and gathering, and even the strength of community belonging (Ahenakew, 2012; Cooke, 2009; Cooke et al., 2008; Drabsch, 2012; Loppie-Reading & Wien, 2009; White, Wingert, et al., 2007). Since the 1970s, the challenges inherent in measuring well-being on subjective and objective levels have been articulated in various forms, ranging from opposing ontological and epistemological approaches to methodological concerns about the ways in which well-being can be empirically assessed and measured over time (Ahenakew, 2012; Cooke et al., 2008; Drabsch, 2012; Ura et al., 2012; White et al., 2000). A review of the literature on well-being frameworks and measurement tools reveals that dimensions and indicators can be limited based on their conceptual design, the people and communities for which they apply, and the lack of available and robust data sources (Cooke et al., 2008; Quinless, 2015). These factors pose considerable challenges for researchers working with Indigenous communities and wanting to utilize these tools in culturally responsive ways. Part of the challenge is recognizing that the conceptualizations used to produce these frameworks and measurement tools are rooted in western knowledge systems that do not adequately reflect Indigenous ways of knowing and seeing the world in a more holistic sense (Loppie-Reading & Wien, 2009; Quinless, 2015).

Over the past three decades, the urbanization of Indigenous peoples has been increasing at a steady rate and is predicted to continue. In 2011, 57 per cent of Indigenous peoples were living in urban areas, up from

54 per cent in 2006 (INAC, 2015b). Indigenous scholars (Corntassel, 2012; Gone, 2011; Kovach, 2005, 2009; Simpson, 2011; Smith, 1999) are aware that Indigenous peoples know who and what they are and thus can make informed lifestyle choices and healthy decisions. Connection to land, culture, and community are key aspects of Indigenous strength, survival, and resurgence (Alfred, 2005; Coulthard, 2014; Simpson, 2017). Engagement in traditional activities and the practice of traditional language are forms of embodied consciousness or grounded normativity (Coulthard, 2014). Research into Indigenous resistance and resurgence has shown that the amount of connection to the land and community that Indigenous peoples maintain through cultural activities and traditional land-based activities helps them cope with the adverse impacts of colonization (Baskin, 2005; Chandler & Lalonde, 1998; Gone, 2011; Gone & Kirmayer, 2010; Kelley et al., 2012; Kirmayer et al., 2011, 2012; Kovach, 2005, 2009; Kral, 2012; Lawson-Te Aho & Liu, 2010; Mundel & Chapman, 2010; Smith, 1999; Wilson & Rosenberg, 2002). However, access to and interactions with traditional lands, cultural activities, communities, language, and Elders, who are often the keepers of traditional knowledge, can be challenging and issues of marginalization due to systemic racism and ethnocentrism that are ever-present in cities for those living a diasporic form of life. Opportunities to live one's identity as an Indigenous person and to cultivate Indigenousness in an urban space can be difficult and may at times seem impossible because many Indigenous cultural practices run counter to dominant western world views. This is further complicated by other socio-economic factors that impact ways of relating to the land that are often prohibitive due to the high costs associated with travelling to one's traditional territory, along with an array of social constraints, such as family and work responsibilities, unemployment, intergenerational trauma, drug and substance abuse, and other barriers (Abele, 2004).

Many Indigenous peoples understand well-being holistically through a balance of the Medicine Wheel, or some rendition of it, that supports the interconnectedness among physical, emotional, spiritual, and mental states of human well-being. The Medicine Wheel with its four quadrants can be linked to the environment, the community, the Nation, and even governance structures (Absolon, 2011; Kelm, 1998; Smith, 1999, 2012). However, wellness as expressed through the FNPOW is also a way of seeing the world that is supported with other concepts embedded in stories, land-based practices, ceremony, art, and songs. The adverse effects of contemporary colonial practices have been identified as a determinant of poor health resulting in lower states of wellness in Indigenous communities (Beavon & Jetté, 2009; Cooke, 2009;

Health Canada, 2002; White, Beavon, et al., 2007; White & Maxim, 2007; White, Wingert, et al., 2007; Wingert, 2011). This has influenced Indigenous peoples' efforts to shape and determine their well-being through the resurgence of Indigenous world views and cultural practices as a strengths-based response to ongoing colonialization, which has acted to systematically deprive Indigenous peoples of their experiences with land, culture, and community. It is strongly recommended that traditional land-based practices through what Coulthard has termed "grounded normativity" (Coulthard, 2014) be seen as a critical component of what it means to be Indigenous. Grounded normativity conceptualizes land as a relationship to Indigenous peoples based in the obligations they have to the land. It is a reciprocal relationship involving all aspects of Indigenous life, culture, and economics (Coulthard, 2014) that, through the Indigenous resurgence movement (Alfred & Corntassel, 2005) and Indigenous research methodologies (Denzin et al., 2008), provides resistance to further dispossession and disconnection by contemporary colonialism.

As Ahenakew (2011; 2012) points out, research has led to the pathologization of Indigenous well-being and post-colonial research practices, in particular, reify deficit states of Indigenous peoples health and wellness (Absolon, 2011, Linklater, 2014; Smith, 1999, 2012). This generates an important question for social researchers focusing on Indigenous issues: "How can western researchers work with Indigenous communities to better understand well-being?" First Nations' relationships with the Canadian government, which are characterized by colonial governance, have negatively influenced their health, resulting in widespread epidemics of infectious diseases, the denigration of Indigenous governing systems, dispossession from the land, dispossession from culture and identity, degradation of health care, and violence against women and children (Aboriginal Affairs Working Group, 2010; Bryce, 1922; Daschuk, 2013; Frideres & Gadacz, 2006; Hutchinson, 2006; Kelm, 1998, Milloy, 1999; Mosby, 2013). A process of decolonizing methodologies makes it possible to generate knowledge supportive of health and wellness outcomes that reflect Indigenous knowledge and teachings. As Anishinaabe scholar and activist Leanne Simpson (2004, p. 377) asserts, "Our knowledge comes from the land, and the destruction of the environment is a colonial manifestation and a direct attack on Indigenous Knowledge and Indigenous nationhood." Indigenous peoples and communities have long experienced exploitation by researchers and there is increasing focus on participatory and decolonizing research processes (Smith, 2006, 2012). There is great value in applying a two-eyed way of seeing health and wellness that bridges aspects of Indigenous knowledge systems and western knowledge systems by holistically examining the determinants of the health and well-being of Indigenous peoples living in urban centres across Canada along physical, mental, spiritual, and emotional dimensions.

Beyond the Western Medical Model and Decolonizing Bodies

What does it mean to decolonize? Decolonization offers different pathways for reconnecting Indigenous peoples with their traditional territories and land/water-based cultural practices. The decolonization process operates at multiple levels and necessitates moving from an awareness of being in struggle to actively engaging in daily practices of resurgence (Coburn, 2015; Corntassel, 2012; Simpson, 2011, 2017). More specifically, it is in those everyday acts of resurgence (Corntassel, 2012) that the scope of the struggle for decolonization is reclaimed by Indigenous peoples. If colonization dispossessed Indigenous peoples from land and culture, "then resurgence is about reconnecting with traditional land-based and water-based cultural practices" (Corntassel, 2012, p. 89). While decolonization and resurgence can be described separately, they are viewed in this book as interrelated actions and strategies that inform pathways to resistance and freedom – everyday decolonization and resurgence practices form the basis of Indigenous health and well-being and applying decolonized research methodologies produces knowledge that supports self-determination.

As Corntassel (2012) points out, "By understanding the overlapping and simultaneous process of decolonization and resurgence, it is possible to better understand how to implement meaningful and substantive community decolonization practices" (p. 99). For example, while working on an Indigenous seed project he states that "initial small-scale efforts might appear to be small but they work towards regenerating the old trade networks between Indigenous communities as well as building healthy relationships by increasing food security and family well-being" (Corntassel, 2012, p. 98). This provides a good example of how everyday acts of community resurgence can support Indigenous people in reclaiming cultural practices that are linked to the land and support them in reclaiming traditions and "liv[ing] responsibly as self-determining nations, Indigenous peoples" (Corntassel, 2012, p. 98). When we reflect on the historical conditions and devastating effects of colonialism on Indigenous family dynamics, states of wellness, and traditional knowledge systems, the importance of maintaining traditional knowledge systems and the role this knowledge plays in decolonization and resurgence is clear. Historically, many traditional Indigenous communities, especially in British Columbia, were considered social networks of related people, called kinships systems or "Keyohs which means resource area" (Brown, 2002, p. 28), which linked family groups to the land with a sense of collective stewardship and ownership over land and also formed the basis of the local economy and sustained "the families belonging to that clan and its sub-clans" (Brown, 2002, p. 28). Traditional communities were social networks based in teachings that engendered collective values such as honour and respect for the land and clan systems that were essential for a balanced way of life (Brown, 2002). Today, the Indigenous freedom movement is based in Indigenous resistance and resurgence in British Columbia and across Canada that supports Indigenous peoples in reconnecting to traditional ways of life as they heal from the destructive struggles against ongoing forces of colonialism.

Mohawk writer, educator, and activist Gerald Taiaiake Alfred (Alfred, 2008) points to what is necessary to make self-determination materialize by laying the intellectual groundwork for the Indigenous resurgence movement that focuses on daily acts of reconnecting Indigenous peoples to the land and cultural ways of life. His standpoint is concerned not with the process through which self-government is negotiated per se, but with the goals and nature of Indigenous government once self-determination has been achieved. He writes:

> It is the central argument of this manifesto that the key to summing and overcoming this crisis is leadership. Leadership will play a crucial role in achieving peace, power and righteousness on the collective level. (Alfred, 2008, p. 13)

Taiaiake Alfred (2008) calls for responsible and ethically guided leadership, which he argues is a critical element in shaping the collective consciousness around the Indigenous Nationhood movement in Canada and globally. Alfred (2008) invites readers to reflect more deeply on issues of reconciliation and how reconciliation will address the impacts of colonization on Indigenous peoples from outside of what he refers to as the "colonial mentality" (Alfred, 2008, p. 94). This means having open conversations about all of the harmful impacts of colonization on Indigenous peoples, which can only begin when people engage in an active process of decolonization of the mind or "the mental state that blocks recognition of the existence or viability of traditional perspectives" (Alfred, 2008, p. 94). At present the public vehicle for this is through the Truth and Reconciliation Framework (TRC, 2015), which is a collective way that Indigenous and non-Indigenous peoples can work collectively to understand the harms inflicted on Indigenous peoples. Hence, colonization, decolonization, self-determination, and

resurgence are all concepts directly linked to reconnection to traditional values and ownership of land (Alfred, 2008). This connection
becomes visible when we understand that "Indigenous community life
is framed by two value systems that are fundamentally opposed. One,
still rooted in traditional teachings, structures social and cultural relations; the other is imposed by the colonial state and structured politics"
(Alfred, 2008, p. 25). Alfred (2008) continues to explain that:

> Indigenous people have successfully engaged Western societies in the first
> stages of a movement to restore their autonomous power and cultural
> integrity in the area of governance. This movement is founded on an ide-
> ology of Native nationalism and a rejection of models of government roo-
> ted in European cultural values. Since the 1980s, little progress has been
> made toward ending the colonial relationship and realizing the ideals of
> Indigenous political thought: respect, harmony, autonomy, and peaceful
> coexistence. (p. 26)

Colonization continues to exist with the legacy of the residential
schools and transgenerational trauma, demoralization by the Indian
Act, and stripping away of Indigenous languages, customs, and ceremonies. All of this has greatly impaired Indigenous peoples' right and
ability to self-govern (Alfred, 2009; Alfred & Corntassel, 2005; Million,
2013; Sayer et al., 2001). While communities have been trying to resolve
these multilayered forms of trauma, the harms that are inflicted by
trauma are ongoing such that:

> Dysfunction, anger and a feeling of helplessness or lack of control impair
> any government that is trying to function and achieve things for the com-
> munity. Community members often focus on the negatives and participate
> in lateral violence. Lateral violence is best described as people, who have
> been colonized then continue to colonize themselves using methods that do
> not promote progress but rather bring others down such as intimidation,
> anger, threats, name-calling and embarrassment. (Sayer et al., 2001, p. 23)

The legacy of the residential school system is ongoing and continues
to impact the health and wellness of Indigenous peoples and their communities. This is apparent in the high number of Indigenous children
who have been removed from their families by child welfare agencies,
overall poor health, and high incarceration rates in Canadian prisons
(Blackstock, 2007; Monchalin, 2016; Nettelbeck, 2016; Sayer et al., 2001).
As the 2015 TRC report (TRC, 2015) outlines, these health gaps are
linked to the legacy of residential schools in such a way that:

The health of generations of Indigenous children was undermined by inadequate diets, poor sanitation and overcrowding and an outbreak of tuberculosis that went untreated. It is reasonable to contend that contemporary Indigenous health status remains far below that of the general population. (p. 132)

Million (2013) has critically observed that trauma is embedded in the era of reconciliation and "Canadian Aboriginal peoples, subjects of a history of colonial violence, are thickly ensconced in the intensities, logics, and languages of trauma, particularly now as they are called on to speak as subjects of 'truth and reconciliation'" (p. 169). Million questions the implications of this trauma-informed reconciliation process for Indigenous peoples where self-determination is vaguely defined and "with the establishment of the TRC, Aboriginal peoples seem to become the subject of a humanitarian project" (Million, 2013, p. 236). She asserts that the TRC and, more specifically, the trauma ethos that is deeply embedded in the TRC, have become a type of regulatory normative violence where Indigenous peoples are regarded as subjects of historical trauma (Million, 2013). This becomes clear when we consider that in 2003, the First Ministers' Accord on Health Care Renewal recognized that Indigenous peoples in Canada were facing serious health issues and there were significant health gaps between Indigenous peoples and non-Indigenous peoples (TRC, 2015). According to the TRC (2015) report, "the federal government has been described as moving backwards on issues of Indigenous health since the signing of the Indian Residential Schools Settlement Agreement" (TRC, 2015, p. 161). To reiterate, the 2015 TRC report reveals that Call to Action Number 65 urges the federal government, through the Social Science and Humanities Research Council and in collaboration with partner academic institutions, to advance the understanding of reconciliation. This means that there is a focus on supporting research in the area of Indigenous health and well-being.

The 2015 TRC Call to Action Number 65 focuses on supporting research partnerships between post-secondary institutions, Indigenous communities, and government organizations as a "necessary structure to document, analyze, and report research findings on reconciliation to a broader audience" (TRC, 2015, p. 242). The 2015 TRC outlines the importance that research will have in the process of reconciliation specific to Call to Action Number 65. It states that:

Research is vital to reconciliation. It provides insights and practical examples of why and how educating non-Indigenous people about the concepts

and practices of reconciliation will contribute to healing and transformative social change. The benefits of research extend beyond addressing the
legacy of residential schools because research on the reconciliation process can inform how Canadian society can mitigate intercultural conflicts,
strengthen civic trust, and build social capacity and practical skills for
long-term reconciliation. (TRC, 2015, p. 242)

What is important to infer from Call to Action Number 65 is that there
is formal recognition that the poor health and well-being of Indigenous
communities is a by-product of the residential school system and that
when validated exclusively by models of western medicine, Indigenous
belief systems and cultural practices are neglected. Indigenous healing is an ongoing journey and includes activities; land-based therapies
such as hunting, gathering, and fishing; and participation in cultural
activities such as drumming, healing circles, sweat lodges, cedar baths,
smudging, and other spiritual ceremonies (Corntassel, 2012; Million,
2013; Monchalin, 2016). Indigenous scholars advocate for using decolonized research practices such as ceremonies and storywork as ways
in which Indigenous peoples can re-establish a connection to the land
and to cultural traditions. It is important to understand how storywork
(Archibald, 2008; Corntassel et al., 2009; Thomas, 2015) is an important
aspect of decolonization and health for Indigenous peoples. For example, Wilson's (2008) work *Research Is Ceremony* offers a paradigm shared
by Indigenous scholars in Canada and Australia on how research relationships between knowledge seekers come to represent Indigenous
reality. Archibald (2008) further explains that Indigenous storytelling is
a gift and an important tool for transforming Coast Salish knowledge
systems through learning and sharing from Elders (Archibald, 2008).
Archibald (2008) suggests that story-based research is critically important for Indigenous peoples and "exemplifies what research should do:
enable people to sit together and talk meaningfully" (p. 81). Using stories is a method and form of healing where problems in community can
be openly discussed.

Health Transformation and Self-determination

Indigenous scholars have advocated that a main component of the Indigenous resurgence movement is to find a balance between living a
socially and economically viable life with environmental sustainability
that is rooted in traditional knowledge systems, laws, and traditions
(Corntassel, 2012; Coulthard, 2014; Simpson, 2011, 2017; Smith, 1999).
Yet, ongoing colonial practices have rendered this near impossible,

especially during the Harper era when, as we have seen outlined in the 2015 TRC, the Government of Canada repeatedly cut funding to critical Indigenous programs such as the Aboriginal Healing Foundation, the National Aboriginal Health Organization, and Health Canada (TRC, 2015). These cuts were accompanied by the Harper government's denial of Canada's colonial past, resulting in "the widening gap between the official state rhetoric of reconciliation and respect and the realities of ongoing, one sided colonial relationship [that] contributes to frustrated expectations" (Denis, 2015, p. 213). These frustrations also contributed to enhanced anger and provided momentum for necessary Indigenous uprisings and acts of self-determination (Denis, 2015). For Indigenous peoples, the spiritual is interconnected with political action but often overlooked in discussions surrounding Indigenous self-determination. As Denis points out, the "spiritual realm is largely neglected by social movements scholars within mainstream non-Indigenous literature" (Denis, 2015, p. 214) but has been ever present during what is commonly known in the Indigenous community as the "8th Fire" with numerous self-determination movement activities across Canada activities and "many Indigenous nations have a prophecy" (Denis, 2015, p. 214).[1] Denis explains this prophecy:

> On December 10, 2012 sacred fires through ceremonial practices were lit across Canada (Turtle Island) to signify Indigenous protests … they creatively used spiritual practices … the round dance quickly became an emblem of the for the movement…Symbols such as the Medicine Wheel and the Two-Row Wampum (or Guswenta), at one a spiritual and political concept, appeared in public discourse. (Denis, 2015. p. 215)

When we think about the Four Directions Medicine Wheel in these ways it becomes clear that Indigenous knowledge is not compartmentalized but exists as an intersection between the balance of the four main dimensions and "all four elements are necessary for an Indigenous self-determination movement to emerge" (Denis, 2015, p. 216). Similarly, the FNHA has created the FNPOW, which is a strengths-based approach to better assist in looking at health and wellness from a holistic lens. This perspective is very important in terms of redefining health from a First Nations perspective and is intended to be used to inform FNHA policy in support of the development of programs and service

---

1 The 8th Fire is an Anishinaabe prophecy that declares now is the time for Aboriginal peoples and the settler community to come together and build the "8th Fire" of justice and harmony. (Denis, 2015).

delivery (FNHA, 2016d). The FNPOW looks at understanding health as a balance of spiritual, emotional, mental, and physical elements and incorporates holistic as well as natural medicines with innovative traditional and contemporary healing "to describe the First Nations Health Authority Vision: Healthy, Self-Determining and Vibrant BC First Nations Children, Families and Communities" (FNHA, 2016d).

Health Governance and the First Nations Health Authority

The British North America Act (1867) resulted in the "division of power (jurisdictions) between the federal and provincial governments" (FNHC, 2011, p. 22). Today, universal health care is provided with the support of funding by the federal government provided to the provinces (FNHC, 2011) and "jurisdictional responsibilities and fiscal struggles between the federal and provincial governments have shaped the creation of the health system in Canada for First Nations" (FNHC, 2011. p.22). The health transfer program was developed primarily by the federal government with minimal consultation with First Nations and in doing so gained supporters and critics (FNHC, 2011). The process of health transfer is rooted in the struggle between funding and control and ownership of First Nations health management and is still an ongoing issue in British Columbia when it comes to the FNHA and the federal and provincial governments. The main tenet supporting health transfer was meant to increase capacity among First Nations in order to deliver mandatory programs and permit First Nations to determine their own program delivery and development.

In 2005, the Transformative Change Accord was signed by the Leadership Council, Government of Canada, and the Province of British Columbia at the First Ministers meeting in Kelowna, whereby:

> The Province of British Columbia and First Nations leaders agreed to enter into a New Relationship guided by principles of trust, recognition and respect for Aboriginal rights and title. The New Relationship focuses on closing the gaps in quality of life between First Nations and other British Columbians. (Government of British Columbia, n.d., p. 2)

In 2006, the Leadership Council and the Province of British Columbia entered into a bilateral agreement to address the health area of the accord and focus on narrowing the health gap. The creation of the First Nations Health Council is identified as the first action item in the Transformative Change Accord. In the accord we see that:

This First Nations Health Plan builds on and supports the First Nations Health Blueprint for British Columbia. It also considers the recommendations of the 2001 report of the Provincial Health Officer entitled The Health and Well-being of Aboriginal People in British Columbia, which was endorsed by First Nations. (Government of British Columbia, n.d., p. 3)

Working in partnership with the FNHA and through participatory action research (PAR) using a mixed methods research approach, my intention is to critically engage in dominant western-based knowledge systems of well-being from a decolonizing standpoint to produce tangible wellness outcomes situated in traditional knowledge systems informed by the FNPOW, the 2012 APS, and the 2011 National Household Survey (NHS). There has been a tendency for Indigenous health initiatives to continue to reflect the values and discourse of the western medical model that are based in a needs-and-pathology paradigm that fails to provide holistic and culturally appropriate wellness solutions to Indigenous peoples. According to Van Uchelen et al. (1997) the question "What makes people strong?" (p. 37) is an important consideration in health research, yet western medical models focus on pathologies that perpetuate deficits and illness (Tuck, 2009). This focuses on "what makes people weak" (Van Uchelen et al., 1997, p. 37). Reading et al. (2007) point to the fact that "First Nations traditional knowledge and healing practices are perhaps the quintessential expressions of a social determinants of health approach" (p. 25). This means that understanding how Indigenous peoples conceptualize wellness and identify their existing strengths and resources offers an alternative approach to the medical model and promotes a strengths-based focus on Indigenous well-being.

The Transformative Change Accord was signed in November 2005 by the Province of British Columbia and the First Nations Leadership Council (FNHC, 2011). As the FNHA began to assume responsibility for the delivery of health services in British Columbia, the organization needed to determine what knowledge must be transferred for accountability but also the terms of measuring progress through program implementation and evaluation (FNHC, 2011). In 2011, the fourth Gathering Wisdom conference offered such an opportunity to move forward and has "been fundamental to shaping the work of the FNHC" (FNHA, 2011, p. 8) with the signing of regional agreements that align healthcare priorities and community health plans and was the place where "BC First Nations were asked to consider and debate an important Resolution to adopt the Consensus Paper, which describes First Nations' vision of a new health governance structure" (FNHA, 2011, p. 8).

The 2012 Gathering Wisdom for a Shared Journey V forum provided an important space for meaningful decision-making processes about what was needed for First Nations communities' health and wellness to move forward in British Columbia but more importantly "First Nations adopted a resolution that allowed for the transition of the interim First Nations Health Authority into the permanent First Nations Health Authority" (FNHA, 2012b, p. 4). A new health and wellness model – the FNPOW – was launched in 2012 at the fifth annual Gathering Wisdom for a Shared Journey conference signalling the first steps of movement away from a deficit-model towards a wellness perspective for BC First Nations (FNHA, 2012b). At that gathering "over 750 representatives including Chiefs, Health Directors, and Provincial and Federal Partners came together to continue talking about our vision for BC First Nations: Healthy Self-Determining and Vibrant BC First Nations Children, Families and Communities" (FNHA, 2012b, p. 3).

The FNHA "is the first of its kind province-wide health authority in Canada" (FNHA, 2016c). In 2013, all of the programs and services that were previously offered and delivered by Health Canada's First Nations Inuit Health Branch, Pacific Region were transferred to the FNHA (HealthlinkBC, 2015). The organization's primary vision is to "transform First Nations and Aboriginal health and well-being for the better" (HealthlinkBC, 2015, p. 1) by implementing a change in health-care provision. This change is inspired by a refusal to accept the continued gap in health outcomes between First Nations and other BC residents. The FNHA is governed on the principles of self-determination and community active engagement in health politics with a specific focus on "increasing First Nations control over decisions relating to health policies, programs and services, and increasing First Nations influence in addressing key health issues with federal and provincial partners" (FNHC, 2011, p. 33). Hence, community engagement has been a fundamental value since the FNHA's inception and serves as the basis of the governance structure for the FNHA (FNHC, 2011).

Gathering Wisdom for a Shared Journey is an ongoing conference series and is considered an important community engagement process. The conference is one of the largest Indigenous health conferences in British Columbia and aims to bring together First Nation peoples with the intent of "shaping a strong and collective vision for First Nation health governance in BC" (FNHC, 2016. p. 1). Community health and well-being are intricately tied to demands for self-determination and "First Nations have been clear that the Gathering Wisdom forum is an important part of the health governance process in BC" (FNHC, 2016. p. 1).

According to the British Columbia Tripartite Framework Agreement on First Nations Health Governance (2011) outlined by Health Canada, the governance structure of the FNHA is comprised of the following (Health Canada, 2011, p. 11):

(a) a First Nations Health Authority (FNHA)
(b) a Tripartite Committee on First Nations Health (Tripartite Committee)
(c) a First Nations Health Council (FNHC)
(d) a First Nations Health Directors Association (FNHDA)

The FNHA is built on the need for self-determination as the basis of a successful health-care delivery model and this model considers traditional as well as modern health knowledges. Specifically, it is stated in the British Columbia Tripartite Framework on First Nations Health Governance that the FNHA shall "incorporate and promote First Nations knowledge, beliefs, values, practices, medicines and models of health and healing into the FN Health Programs" (Health Canada, 2011, p. 11). The FNHA's purpose is to narrow the health gap between First Nations and other residents of British Columbia through community engagement processes and to "plan, design, manage, deliver and fund the delivery of FN Health Programs" (Health Canada, 2011, p. 11).

The FNHA is governed by an experienced board of directors comprised of ten members collectively holding experience in areas of "First Nation health, community development, financial management and politics, all at various levels of government" (FNHA, 2016b, n.p.).[2] The Board "provides leadership and oversight for the activities of the FNHA" (FNHA, 2016b, n.p.). Initially, the FNHA was created in conjunction with the First Nations Health Council to provide support services mandated by two health agreements collectively known as the Health Plans (FNHA, 2016a). These are (1) the Transformative Change Accord: First Nations Health Plan, 2006 and (2) the Tripartite First Nations Health Plan, 2007. Additionally, FNHA follows the Framework Agreement, which builds on previous agreements represented by signing the Transformative Change Accord (2005), the Transformative Change Accord: First Nations Health Plan (2006), the First Nations Health Plan Memorandum of Understanding (2006), the Tripartite

---

2 In 2016, board members included Lydia Hwitsum (Chair), Jason Calla (Secretary Treasurer) and Marion Colleen Erickson (Vice Chairperson), Helen Joe, Dr. Elizabeth Whynot, Jim Morrison, Norman Thompson, David Goldsmith, and Graham Whitmarsh (FNHA, 2016b).

First Nations Health Plan (2007), the Basis for a Framework Agreement on First Nation Health Governance (2010), and the British Columbia Tripartite Framework Agreement on First Nation Health Governance (2011) (FNHA, 2016a). The signing of these agreements initiates forward-looking plans that have guided the transfer of responsibility for the design and implementation of all federally funded health programs and services for BC First Nations from Health Canada to the FNHA in British Columbia (FNHA, 2016a, 2016e; FNHC, 2011).

FNHA has parted from the status quo in terms of First Nations delivery of health-care services and programs and has set forth an innovative plan for health and wellness in British Columbia. This is a formidable task and is the mandate of the FNHA together with working in collaboration with federal and provincial governments and the previously stated agreements are ways that the FNHA is intending to close the close the health gap and transform health governance for First Nations in British Columbia (FNHA, n.d.). The Relationship Agreement emphasizes the "sound partnership sought by the Parties – a partnership based on shared values and understanding of our collective and respective roles, responsibilities, and accountabilities" (FNHA, n.d., p. 3). It outlines roles, mandates components to self-government, and sets shared values between the FNHA, the First Nations Health Council (FNHC), and the First Nations Health Directors Association. According to the FNHA Relationship Agreement report (FNHA, n.d, pp. 5–6), there are six shared values among the three partners: respect, discipline, relationships, culture, excellence, and fairness. Operating principles, which are "ideals underlying how we seek to interact with one another, our partners, our communities and beyond" (FNHA, 2013a, p. 12) have also been developed by FNHA. The operating principles from the FNHA Annual Report: 2012–2013 are summarized as follows:

> The FNHA will operate in a manner that emphasizes a wellness philosophy that is based in First Nations teachings … an emphasis on being the best human beings we can be … leadership by example and being an organization that models wellness … being a learning organization, not leaving people behind, implementing First Nations traditional knowledge and offering service delivery driven by community engagement and a business approach that encourages sustainability, integrity, efficiency and innovation in service and program delivery. (FNHA, 2013a, p. 12)

The decolonization of research methodologies has been a leading research priority for over two decades (Smith, 2012) and is widely recognized as being emancipatory and inciting positive social change because "it engages with imperialism and colonialism at multiple levels" (Smith, 2012, p. 21). The objective of a decolonizing approach is not to "discard all theory or Western knowledge" (Smith, 1999, p. 39); rather, decolonizing methodologies draw from existing knowledge and bridge western and Indigenous knowledge systems. This is also necessary for two-eyed seeing. Decolonizing research advocates a *re*-searching of knowledge using critical engagement with dominant discourse that builds on Indigenous knowledge and requires a change in conceptualizations of the research process and a focus on the development of new paradigms and different ways of thinking about what it means to be Indigenous (Corntassel, 2012; Kovach, 2005, 2009; Simpson, 2011, 2017; Smith 1999, 2012). As previously discussed, the FNHA advocates for a strengths-based approach to health research, which means making a concerted effort to focus on what is working well within Indigenous communities as opposed to continually exemplifying community problems and health deficits; the latter has been overemphasized in western medical models. A strengths-based approach has grown from Indigenous resilience research emerging from developmental psychology and psychiatry in recent years (Kirmayer et al., 2011). This book supports a strengths-based approach to well-being research and demonstrates that, as a form of social capital, well-being can be a resource utilized by Indigenous peoples to invest in and experience enhanced wellness and to strengthen their lives and local communities. This will require a decolonization of Indigenous bodies as a collective given the connection of Indigenous bodies to poor health due to the forces of colonization.

To be healthy and whole an Indigenous person needs to be centred, which means to be balanced between one's self, other humans, and the natural environment. As stated earlier, an important part of the FNHA mandate is to incorporate First Nations' cultural knowledge, beliefs, values, and models of healing into the re-design and delivery of health programs. It contains ideas that are not new to BC First Nations but come from traditional teachings, healers, and natural medicines. The FNPOW creates a wellness environment that is used to support existing traditional approaches to health and "is intended to serve as a starting point for discussion by First Nations communities on what they conceptualize as a vision of wellness for themselves and the FNHA" (FNHA, 2016d). The FNPOW is used to create a shared understanding of what health and wellness mean in BC First Nations communities that is supported by the FNHA and shared with partner organizations, the federal government, and the general public.

4

Social Capital Theory, Health Indicators, and Indigenous Communities

Empirical research into the association between social capital and health has provided strong support, with testable hypotheses and interpretive results, for considering social capital as a health determinant (Robson & Sanders, 2009). This chapter considers the relationships that occur across individual and community levels of well-being that emerge in the urban landscape. The focus of this chapter is to provide an overview of social capital and to offer insight into how this theoretical framework will support its application to health and wellness within Indigenous communities. To fully appreciate the utility of social capital as one eye in a two-eyed seeing approach to research methods, decolonization, and Indigenous health, it will be useful to review the conceptual frameworks and measurement tools that have been developed as composite measures of well-being since the 1970s by various countries, organizations, and groups. The chapter will also outline many of the frameworks and indicators recently developed to measure Indigenous wellness and its associated attributes in Canada with an introduction to the FNPOW. The focus here is to provide an overview of social capital and to offer insight into how this theoretical framework will support the ways in which it can be applied to health and wellness within Indigenous communities. The objective of this chapter will be to explain how social capital acts as a resource that is owned by the individual as part of their internal capacity but also as a contributing factor that makes up community capacity.

Historical Overview: Bourdieusian Social Capital and Health Status

The concept of social capital articulated by Pierre Bourdieu provides a solid theoretical framework and the concept has been used and further developed in studies of well-being. Social capital analysis is important for policymakers and developmental practitioners to better address issues surrounding Indigenous health and wellness. Bourdieusian analysis emphasizes three forms of capital: economic, cultural, and social. In his book *Distinction: A Social Critique of the Judgement of Taste,* Pierre Bourdieu (1984) suggests that western societies consist of hierarchical class structures that are stratified and differentiated according to the amount and combination of forms of the capital that members of each social class accumulate and "there is a strong correlation between social positions and the dispositions of the agents who occupy them" (Bourdieu, 1984, p. 110). The objectified forms of capital can be regarded as a type of raw material (Moore, 2012) and the conversion of these three forms of capital function to structure and reproduce the society's objective hierarchical structures and systems of stratification as well as the person's subjective understanding of their place within these structures and systems or their class (Moore, 2012; Moore et al., 2005). For Bourdieu, society's objective structures were embodied within individuals and expressed through their bodily disposition and health status as signalled by an "increased spending on health and beauty care and clothing, a slight increase on cultural and leisure activities" (Bourdieu, 1984, p. 180). In this way, an individual's class disposition and health distinguished the individual from members in other class strata and in so doing reinforced the social order. Bourdieu was one of the first to articulate the negative nature of social capital. He conceptualizes it as an upper-class resource of distinction that functions to give access to resources for upper-class members while excluding access to resources for lower-class members and that "tastes in food also depend on the idea each class has of the body and of the effects of food on the body, that is, on its strength, health and beauty" (Bourdieu, 1984, p. 190).

For Bourdieu (1984), the structure of the social world is related to all forms of capital, not only those strictly associated with economic theory but social capital as a relational resource. As a relational resource, social capital is composed of a variety of different elements, which include social networks, social norms and values, trust, and shared resources (Bourdieu, 1984; Bourdieu & Wacquant, 1992; Moore, 2012). Bourdieu relates social capital to actual or potential resources within a social structure, which then supports each of its members – "for example, the financial managers of the largest firms, who are almost all Sciences or HEC [hautes études commerciales] graduates, who possess a large social capital (family connections, their respective 'old-boy networks') often belong to clubs" (Bourdieu, 1984, p. 310). Bourdieu links social capital as a resource associated to the possession of a network of relationships of mutual acquaintances to be a type of conversion between networks. To elaborate, Veenstra (2009) also points out that transmutations of social capital refer to the process whereby one form of capital is converted into another, and that "it appears that social capital comes in multiple forms, adopting various meanings in Canadian social space and appearing in different conversion processes with economic and cultural capital" (Veenstra, 2009, p. 73).

Bourdieu theorized capital conversions extensively and empirically investigates them in *Distinction: A Social Critique of the Judgement of Taste* (1984). He argues that structure is not an object that is initially visible to the observer, since analysis always proceeds by considering the various effects of this structure. Thus, the researcher must reconstruct this structure and its symbolic space within their position in society by considering the relationships between these effects. In reconstructing the habitus, the researcher must take into consideration "homologous to their own position in the dominant class" the conditions of existence that manifest in practices (Bourdieu, 1984). To reconstruct the structure of practices, Bourdieu (1984) argues that we must break from linear thinking:

> [The] structural causality of a network of factors is quite irreducible to the cumulated effects of the set of linear relationships ... through each of the factors is exerted the efficacy of all the others, and the multiplicity of determinations leads not to indeterminacy but to over-determination. ... One of the difficulties of sociological discourse lies in the fact that, like all language, it unfolds in strictly linear fashion, whereas, to escape oversimplification and one-sidedness, one ought to be able to recall at every point the whole network of relationships found there and attribute analytic primacy to factors which have the greatest functional weight. (p. 107)

Bourdieu (1984) suggests these factors consist primarily of the volume and composition of economic, social, cultural, and symbolic forms of capital. Moreover, the volume and composition of capital should always be assessed in relation to the field of contention, which determines the variability in the functional weight of capital:

> Capital is a social relation, for example, an energy which only exists and only produces its effects in the field in which it is produced and reproduced. Each of the properties attached to class govern its value and efficacy by the specific laws of each field. (Bourdieu, 1984, p. 113)

The social scientist must also take change, as it relates to the volume and composition of capital, into consideration. The structure of the habitus is the product of both inculcation and stability; this could include, for example, family, experiences, conditions of existence, and the effects of social trajectory – "that is, the effects of social rise or decline on dispositions and opinions" (Bourdieu, 1984, p. 111). Bourdieu (1984) further argues that:

> the habitus, an objective relationship between two objectivities, enables an intelligible and necessary relation to be established between practices and a situation, the meaning of which is produced by the habitus through categories of perception, and appreciation that are themselves produced by an observable social condition. (p. 101)

This break from conventional linear thinking Bourdieu outlines has been an invitation for sociologists to conceptualize ways of applying social capital analysis using more innovative methods for surpassing simple linear relationships between factors. As Heck and Thomas (2015) point out:

> Research strategies for dealing with the complexity of the multilevel, or contextual, features of organizations have been somewhat limited historically and researchers did not always consider the implications of the assumptions they made about measuring variables at their natural level, or moving them from one level to another through aggregation or disaggregation. (p. 3)

Contemporary analytical strategies of estimating random coefficients models using covariance structure modelling make it possible to estimate both fixed and random effects, which enables research models to aggregate and disaggregate data. With estimating fixed and random effects, it is possible to translate the general linear model into multilevel equation modelling (Heck & Thomas, 2015). For example, we are no longer restricted when we use the analysis of covariance that the relationships between our covariant are the same across different groups of our predictor variables because multilevel modelling can model variability through random effects estimation. There has been a shift in statistical techniques and a move away from oversimplified models "in examining phenomena that entail the nesting of individuals within higher-order groups" (Heck & Thomas, 2015, p. 7). Knowing these techniques has created a shift in what is possible analytically, which in turn can influence how we think theoretically and conceptually.

Bourdieu (1984) notes that our fundamental experience of the social world is one based on misrecognition, not one predicated on a unitary or factional consciousness. The habitus, by its imputing of values and qualifiers on objects and objective relations, generates differential life-styles that are not only opposed to one another but also predicated on misrecognition. For Bourdieu, structure is not initially visible to the observer because analysis always proceeds by taking into account the various effects of this structure. The researcher has to reconstruct this structure and its symbolic space by considering the relationships between these effects and "to do this, one must return to the practice-unifying and practice-generating principle, i.e., class habitus, the inter-nalized form of class conditions and of the conditionings it entails" (Bourdieu, 1984, p. 101). Moreover, the habitus generates a systemic and structured relation to the world, varying, of course, by class. In Bourdieu's own words, "the practices of all agents of the same class, owe the stylistic affinity which makes each of them a metaphor of any of the others to the fact that they are the product of transfers of the same schemes of actions, from one field to another" (Bourdieu, 1984, p. 173).

Bourdieu further suggests that the equilibrium between supply and demand is not predicated on an abstract economistic logic but is, rather, constituted in two independent but related fields of experience: con-sumption and production. Consumption is but a manifestation of the tastes of consumers, which is an expression of the habitus (Bourdieu, 1984) itself manifested in embodied dispositions and shaped by the appropriation of objectified culture. By virtue of the class structure, Bourdieu (1984) suggests that actors do not move randomly within the social structure; rather, their life paths are determined by restrictions and inertia, which are an outcome of the convergence between sub-jective dispositions and objective conditions. Bourdieu notes that, as objective conditions change and as families and actors try to increase or maintain their assets, so do the subjective orientations of classes. These changes represent strategies, "conscious or unconscious tendencies" (Bourdieu, 1984, p. 106) that function to maintain class structure, which operates on relational distinctions. Bourdieu (1984) argues:

> [These] strategies depend, first, on the volume and composition of capital to be reproduced; and, secondly, on the state of the instruments of repro-duction (inheritance law and custom, the labour market, the educational system, etc.), which itself depends on the state of the power relations between classes. (p. 125)

Classes can strategically convert one type of capital to another and change the asset structure of classes, which is an important aspect of Bourdieusian analysis when applied to Indigenous well-being especially when multilevel estimation methods are used to account for conceptualizations of social capital as both an individual-level and contextual-level resource. Bourdieu (1984) further notes that the variable strategies implemented by the classes either to maintain or change their position necessarily result in a displacement of the class structure (and the distribution of the assets at stake). However, this change is cancelled out by the various strategies that are implemented by other classes. This reveals an interesting relationship between stability and change – that class structure changes and, in doing so, preserves itself. The relationship between stability and change is thus coextensive:

> It can be seen how naïve it is to claim to settle the question of "social change" by locating "newness" or "innovation" in a particular site in social space ... to characterize a class as "conservative" or "innovating" ... by tacit recourse to an ethical standard which is necessarily situated socially, produces a discourse which states little more than the site it comes from, because it sweeps aside ... the field of struggles. (Bourdieu, 1984, p. 156)

Later, Bourdieu (1986) further pioneered the capital resource discussion by presenting three common forms of capital: economic, cultural, and social. Woolcock (2001) began to elaborate different roles of social capital because "in order to accommodate the range of outcomes associated with social capital, it is necessary to recognize the multidimensional nature of its sources" (p. 10). *Bonding* social capital involves informal networks such as family, friends, and neighbours, while *bridging* social capital involves more distant networks such as colleagues and associates. Bonding and bridging are essentially considered horizontal relationships (Levitte, 2004). Important for policymakers and developmental practitioners is the recognition that social capital also comes in vertical form, as *linking* social capital. Woolcock's (2001) work has supported an elaboration of social capital that moves beyond the notion of the "good marketing" aspect of social capital and addresses "the hype surrounding social capital, like any 'product,' would have collapsed under its own weight long ago if there wasn't a sufficiently rigorous empirical foundation on which it was built, and if a broad constituency of people didn't 'buy it'" (p. 13). The concept of social capital articulated by Bourdieu (1984) has provided a solid theoretical basis and the concept of social capital has been used in a variety of interdisciplinary studies of well-being. For example, empirical research into the association between social capital and health has provided strong support for considering social capital as a health determinant, with testable hypotheses and interpretive results (Robson & Sanders, 2009). It is with this in mind that the concept of social capital is useful for non-Indigenous practitioners in understanding aspects of individual and community well-being with testable hypotheses for Indigenous peoples (First Nations) living in urban centres across Canada, which will be discussed in the following section.

Social Capital Analysis and Applied Social Research

There is increasing acknowledgment that social capital is an important determinant of health and well-being. Specifically, the concept can be applied in an empirical context to provide evidence regarding the direction and strength of the linkages between various aspects of health and well-being through the use of multilevel statistical modelling, which will be discussed in more detail in chapter 5. A number of Canadian studies have applied social capital in diverse areas of community well-being and in the context of Indigenous communities (Canadian Council on Learning, 2007; Clarkson et al., 1992). For example, in 2007, the Assembly of First Nations described social capital in the context of understanding health policy through "achieving a more wholistic approach to Aboriginal well-being" (Reading et al., 2007, p. 24) and the First Nations Social Cohesion Project of the Population Studies Centre at the University of Western Ontario explored through a series of papers how variations among forms of capital and cohesiveness within First Nations communities generate different outcomes at a population level (Maxim et al., 2003; White et al., 2000; White, Beavon, et al., 2007; White & Maxim, 2007; White, Wingert, et al., 2007). Mignone and O'Neil (2005b), in their study of three First Nations communities, further suggest that social capital is specific to First Nations communities in terms of the extent to which local resources are socially invested and also the extent to which the community possesses diverse networks to share and expand these social investments. The concepts of bonding, bridging, and linking social capital are common in the literature on community aspects of social capital (Lofors & Sundquist, 2007; Mignone. 2009; Mignone & O'Neil, 2005a, 2005b; White, Beavon, et al., 2007; White & Maxim, 2007; Whitley et al., 2005). The findings of the study conducted by Mignone and O'Neil (2005b) in three First Nations communities showed that "the social capital of a community is assessed through a combination of its bonding (relations within the community), bridging (relations with other communities), and linkage (relations with formal institutions) dimensions" (p. 27). But the issue I raise is that colonization has an ongoing impact on well-being and has deprived Indigenous peoples and communities of all three forms of capital and constructed socio-political fields that have situated Indigenous peoples in subaltern locations.

Reading et al. (2007) prepared a report on behalf of the Assembly of First Nations that described social capital in the context of understanding health policy through a more holistic lens to policymakers with the aim to improve health by:

> integrating Indigenous knowledge systems into advanced health policy development and research in an effort to combine scientific excellence with community relevance from project design to analysis, interpretation of results and translation of knowledge to policy makers with the aim to improve health. (p. 35)

In addition, the First Nations Social Cohesion Project of the Population Studies Centre at the University of Western Ontario produced a series of papers to explore how variations among forms of capital and cohesiveness within First Nations communities generate different outcomes at the population level (Maxim et al., 2003; White et al., 2000). Social capital is considered a useful concept to better understand individual and community levels of well-being as a form of investment or community capacity and the researchers point out that "just as we see a process of building social capital we can see that certain processes depreciate social capital. An example would be migration" (White et al., 2000, p. 12).

Social Capital Theory and Colonization

We are, in Marx's terms, "an ensemble of social relations" (Marx, 1978) and we live our lives at the core of the intersection of unequal social relations based on hierarchically interrelated structures that, together, define the historical specificity of the capitalist modes of production and reproduction and underlie their observable manifestations (Marx, 1978). When we regard the social capital of health and well-being from the political economy of health perspective, it is strikingly clear that there are systems of inequality (Loppie-Reading & Wien, 2009; Reading et al., 2007). It is challenging to articulate the ways in which common interests, ideologies, politics, and experiences based on class location and socio-economic status are different and similar among groups of Indigenous peoples. In turn, people sharing the same class location, or similar socio-economic characteristics within a class, are themselves further divided along multiple axes such as gender, age (Darnovsky et al., 1995), and Indigenous identity.

While the relationship between structural changes, class formations, and political consciousness is more complex than what classical Marxism would suggest, Bourdieu's multiple forms of capital have helped to shed light on some of these issues. Bourdieu's (1984) work on culture and forms of capital can broaden our understanding of social class in relation to Indigenous health and wellness when we conceive of health as a form of capital and investment. For example, Bourdieu's concept of habitus, which is defined as a set of dispositions, reflexes, and forms of behaviour people acquire through acting in society, can be used to reflect the different positions people have in society (Crossley, 2003). This could be, for example, whether they are brought up in a middle-class environment within a large census metropolitan area (CMA) like Vancouver, British Columbia, or in a working-class suburb such as a census agglomeration (CA) area like Duncan, British Columbia.

The work of Bourdieu (1984) offers a cogent conceptual framework for extending the notion of resources beyond economic and social capital to include symbolic and cultural forms and in doing so creates a moment when subjective orientations are not in line with objective realities. In such instances, the doxic practices (naturalizing beliefs and opinion) are suspended and the actor, in a self-reflexive manner, reconstructs their habitus so as to align their subjective position with objective conditions and doxa has "a further epistemological dimension, which in turn leads to the need for greater reflexivity on the parts of its agents" (Deer, 2012, p. 115). This description helps to articulate how the possession of cultural and symbolic capital affects health and wellness and is useful to consider when Indigenous peoples participate in wellness activities such as hunting, gathering, arts and crafts, and making traditional clothing and footwear. As Crossley (2003) points out, "Class-based cultural advantages are passed from parents to children through the habitus, but as pre-reflective and habitual acquisitions they are generally misrecognized within the school system as 'natural talents' and are rewarded 'appropriately'" (p. 43). This all relates to how class can engender symbolic and cultural forms (Crossley, 2003).

From this standpoint, class relations remain an important frame of reference for making sense of people's everyday lives in such a way that everydayness becomes a way of uncovering aspects of social capital. As previously discussed in this chapter, the effects of colonization and western approaches to understanding health and well-being such as the western medical model, the CWB, and general attitudes of health researchers have resulted in ongoing health problems for Indigenous peoples with few improvements in these health conditions over time.

When we think about social capital as a commodity, the question that emerges is "Who benefits from the continuity of Indigenous people's poor health?" The proposed answer is that many non-Indigenous groups benefit, especially those groups that control and influence the distribution of scarce resources across Indigenous communities. This becomes apparent when we consider the current battles over land and access to resources occurring in the Province of British Columbia among Indigenous communities, provincial governments, and large multinational corporations.

For example, Wilkes (2015) has collected newspaper articles and Indigenous-focused media to create an Indigenous Resistance data-set that tracks Indigenous resistance struggles and in doing so points out that the proposed Enbridge Northern Gateway pipeline created numerous Indigenous resistance events against a multimillion-dollar advertising campaign that tried to sell the project to First Nations and the non-Indigenous public (Wilkes, 2015). The propaganda touted "the Project" would improve the social and economic lives of Indigenous peoples living in the area with long-term economic benefits to the communities along the pipeline corridor route (Northern Gateway, 2016, n.p.). The Indigenous peoples of this area were told that in compensation for the project one of the main benefits that Enbridge would offer was an investment in their skills training. At the same time, Enbridge (Northern Gateway, 2016) stated that:

> Northern Gateway and First Nations and Métis communities are building a true partnership, one that includes environmental stewardship and monitoring, shared ownership of 33%, a joint governance structure and enhanced benefits of $2 billion for First Nations and Métis communities, providing long-term economic prosperity for generations of First Nations and Métis peoples. (n.p.)

In this scenario, we can see where the capital gains are to be had and it is not with Indigenous peoples who are told they will benefit from the proposed Enbridge project. How will Indigenous peoples' wellness from colonialism be restored, their family lives enhanced, their children's sense of happiness secured, and the sacredness of their lands that they use for ceremonies be protected through promises of job skills and training? As noted by Taiaike Alfred, "to focus solely on the socioeconomic status of Indigenous peoples is to perpetuate an assimilationist model whereby Indigenous peoples are slotted in to the capitalist wage economy" (as cited in Wilkes, 2015, p. 118). This entire scenario is highly problematic.

The concept of interconnectedness is fundamental to Indigenous world views and an extraction of resources from the land for purely financial gain runs counter to these world views. This type of social capital framework assumes that all groups of people within a society have the same goals as well as similar stakes in the process. Social capital is a useful concept that can be applied to individual and community levels of well-being as a form of investment related to economic development for Indigenous peoples and communities.

As a process of domination and land dispossession, colonialism has proven destructive to the peoples of the world who have experienced colonization. As discussed in chapter 2, Indigenous peoples in Canada suffered severe impacts of colonization observed through dispossession from their lands, languages, cultural practices, knowledge systems, kinship networks, communities, families, and Indigenous identity. Western biomedical models of health and wellness with their focus on diagnosis and treatment have further impacted Indigenous people negatively by reducing Indigenous peoples and communities to a series of health problems that need fixing (Knibb-Lamouche, 2012) and by governments who put forward policies aimed at solving the "Indian problem." Colonization has negatively impacted all forms of social capital for Indigenous peoples at the individual and community levels, and social capital models used in the future must address systemic structures of colonialism. There are ways in which social capital can be used to understand individual and community Indigenous wellness, as Ledogar and Fleming (2008a) suggest in their work on resilience:

> Social capital, as an asset or a resource for resilience, can be a characteristic of the community or the individual. As an individual asset, social capital consists of a person's relationships to available social resources. As a characteristic of communities, it consists of attributes such as trust, reciprocity, collective action, and participation. Closely related to community social capital is the concept of collective efficacy. Some social networks, however, can be violent, repressive, bigoted, or otherwise destructive. (p. 1)

Ledogar and Fleming (2008a) further suggest that individual and community resilience can be linked to both positive and negative forms of capital when we "recognize that individuals can be resilient even if the communities they live in have low or even negative social capital" (p. 1) that could be in the form of low levels of education or low proportions of people who speak an Indigenous language. Using social capital to understand determinants of Indigenous health and wellness means that when we think about health it is necessary to start to broaden our definitions to include the physical, mental, emotional, and spiritual well-being of individuals and attempt to do so at the community level as well. The constant discourse of the western medical model and other failed attempts at understanding Indigenous health and wellness in Canada, such as the CWB, serve to model "over" Indigenous peoples and emphasize inadequacy, which disconnects Indigenous peoples from their own identities in a manner like past oppressive policies of colonization and assimilation. In lieu of this, several scholars are now exploring social capital in different ways that focus on the individual and the community through a combination of relations and networks.

The "social capital of a First Nations community is understood and assessed through a combination of its internal community relations (bonding), its intercommunity ties (bridging), and the relations the community has with formal institutions (linking)" (Mignone, 2003, p. 32). In a later article, Mignone (2009) further describes a community-based research project, which she conducted through the University of Manitoba and several First Nations communities in Manitoba, that developed culturally appropriate measurement tools and a conceptual framework to measure social capital for these First Nations communities. Social capital for a community was defined as the degree to which the community resources were socially invested, there was a sense of trust, and reciprocity was practised, whereby:

> *Bonding* social capital refers to internal community relations. *Bridging* social capital is essentially a horizontal notion, implying connections between societies, communities or groups, i.e., the inter-community ties. *Linking* social capital refers to a vertical dimension, i.e., the relations with formal institutions beyond the community. (Mignone, 2009, p. 108)

Mignone and O'Neil (2005b) also describe another social capital project where they developed a conceptual framework of social capital for First Nations communities through a comprehensive literature review and ethnographic fieldwork, and conclude that:

> Social capital characterizes a First Nation community based on the degree that its resources are socially invested; that it presents a culture of trust, norms of reciprocity, collective action, and participation; and that it possesses inclusive, flexible, and diverse networks. Social capital of a community is assessed through a combination of its bonding (relations within

the community), bridging (relations with other communities), and linkage (relations with formal institutions) dimensions. (p. 27)

As these studies have indicated, what makes social capital particularly useful when applied to Indigenous communities is that it can be either negative or positive; as a resource in the context of well-being, this offers insight into how social capital influences community capacity. For example, Salée (2006) states that a breakdown in social cohesion within communities may degrade enterprising vitality through a loss of community-based social capital (e.g., trust, bonding, support) but also that "society-wide increases in social capital (and, implicitly, in social cohesion) are thus more likely to have a strongly positive effect on well-being and the general quality of life" (p. 7), while O'Brien et al. (2005) suggest that reconciling Indigenous bonding and bridging social capital is a difficult issue and may be extremely important in regards to addressing economic development and global issues of inequality. Building social capital ties within Indigenous communities "requires building social capital ties" (O'Brien et al., 2005, p. 1050) that can be linked to the larger mainstream community but doing so can be challenging.

Putnam's (1995) ideas on social capital suggest that "life-networks, norms, and trust ... enable participants to act together more effectively to pursue shared objectives" (p. 664). This extends the idea that building and maintaining external bridging and bonds is a way in which social capital is a precursor to influencing positive change in urban Indigenous communities through social cohesion (Putnam, 1995). The ideas of bridging and bonds have been used to explore the relationship between social resources and health. For example, a neighbourhood study by Kim et al. (2006) examines the association between community-level social capital and individual-level self-reported poor health in 40 communities in the United States. The findings reveal that, after adjusting for individual-level factors and community-level variables, community-bonding social capital and community-bridging social capital are associated with significantly lower odds of self-reported poor health. The findings of this study support the relationship between neighbourhood resources and health status. The authors conclude that "interventions and policies that leverage community bonding and bridging social capital might serve as means of population health improvement" (Kim et al., 2006, p. 116).

As another example, *The Harvard Project on American Indian Economic Development* founded in 1987 through Harvard University aims to understand and foster the conditions under which sustained, self-determined social and economic development are achieved among American Indian Nations.[1] The main findings of the project revolve around four main tenets when it comes to economic and social development: sovereignty, institutions, culture, and leadership (Simeone, 2007). For example, when Indian Nations make their own decisions about what development approaches to take, they exercise sovereignty over their own affairs. For development to take hold, assertions of sovereignty must be backed by capable institutions of governance and leaders who introduce new knowledge and experiences in nation-building processes (Cornell & Kalt, 1998). The work emerging out of the Harvard project has been extended to the Indigenous communities in urban centres across Canada as a way of designing models of tribal-owned operations. There is an emphasis on entrepreneurial initiatives to enhancing the tribal economy that supports the view that a "nation-building approach requires new ways of thinking about economic development" (Cornell et al., 1998, p. 8). As Peters (2009) also points out, when the four main components are in place, successful economies are based in legitimate, culturally grounded institutions of self-government. For example, urban centres will differ in their opportunities and challenges and, in their attempts to achieve sovereignty, "there may be more opportunities for 'institutional completeness' in some urban areas because the large numbers of Aboriginal people can support a variety of initiatives" (Peters, 2009, n.p.).

As an individual resource, social capital consists of a person's relationships to available social resources such as education, training, and employment opportunities. While community social capital which has been characterized by Putnam (1993, 1995) and is sometimes called "ecological social capital" (Whitley & McKenzie, 2005), it consists of a community's capacity and its connection to available resources, which could include social services, affordable housing, healing centres, and employment through industry.

A study conducted by Hodge et al. (2011) yielded important insights into the concept of wellness among American Indians and the role story-telling plays in defining well-being. The results showed that among many tribes, the concept of wellness is defined as the physical, mental/emotional, spiritual, and environmental traits that together form

---

1 The Harvard Project focuses on research, education, and the administration of a tribal governance awards program. The Harvard Project collaborates with the Native Nations Institute for Leadership, Management and Policy at the University of Arizona. The Harvard Project is affiliated with the Harvard University Native American Program at Harvard University. See www.hks.harvard.edu

balance and harmony in life through stories. The failure of any or all parts of balance in life (wellness) appears to be closely tied to general health status and was shown in this study to be associated with health conditions; "storytelling was used in the project as an educational and cultural tool to motivate Native people toward healthier behavior" (Hodge et al., 2011, p. 2).

What these studies reveal is that social capital is a useful concept for working with Indigenous communities provided it is conceptualized by those Indigenous communities, as is the case with the FNPOW. Social capital is a relational and transformative concept that is embedded in cultural meanings and symbols and can be valuable in understanding and improving Indigenous health and well-being at the individual and community levels (Baum, 2007; Ledogar & Fleming, 2008b; Mignone, 2003, 2009; Mignone & O'Neil, 2005b; Veenstra, 2009).

As discussed in chapter 1, the good life or Mino-Biimaaddiziwin can be interpreted as a form of social capital that reflects the network of institutions and organizations within a community to deliver programs and services. It is also the capacity of citizens within a community to engage in these activities offered through these programs and services (Hill & Cooke, 2014; Newhouse & Fitzmaurice, 2012). But what are the indicators to measure and assess these forms of social capital and, in the context of Indigenous well-being and social capital, who decides which indicators are included and which are excluded? There has been a plethora of research work dedicated to exploring the extent to which socially cohesive communities create bonds of trusting relationships that act as bridging processes where individuals and institutions can participate in community development projects (Carli, 2012; Chataway, 2002; Côté, 2012; Hill & Cooke, 2014; Mignone & O'Neil, 2005a, 2005b; Newhouse & Fitzmaurice, 2012).

Well-being is a multifaceted concept and the ways in which it is conceptualized and the measures used to define and implement it have not been consistent over time, partly due to the fact that "well-being means different things to different people at different times" (Quinless, 2015, p. 86). A closer examination reveals that current research trends reflect a shift in how Indigenous well-being is conceptualized and recognize that indicators of well-being operate on a number of subjective and objective dimensions at individual, family, community, and even state levels (Chretien, 2010). This contributes to the difficulty of defining and measuring well-being, and the task to do so requires an understanding of both objective and subjective indicators, of the extent to which they are interconnected, and of how they change over time. For example, subjective measures include individual health status, intimate relationships, sense of personal safety, and a sense of connection to a community, while objective measures focus on broad categories and include factors such as the economy, the environment, social conditions, governance, business, and national security (Cummins et al., 2008; Richmond et al., 2007).

Moving beyond the GDP: Social and Economic Indicators of Well-being

It is widely recognized that well-being is a complex concept with interconnected factors that operate on many subjective and objective levels for Indigenous peoples and is linked with other holistic aspects related to states of health along physical, mental, social, and spiritual dimensions. This holistic understanding of well-being is also supported by the World Health Organization's definition of human health as stated in the principles set out in the preamble to its constitution: "a state of complete physical, mental and social well-being and not merely the absence of disease and infirmity" (WHO, 2006, p. 1). This holistic dimension is the outcome of a shift in thinking that started in the 1970s when there was a move away from reliance on conventional economic measures such as GDP and GNP as the main indicators of progress and development. As Haque (2004) points out:

> No matter how parochial, superficial, and misleading the GNP measure may be, it has been effectively used by development experts and agencies in stereotyping postcolonial societies, certifying their ranks in global economic order, imposing on them the inappropriate development policies and strategies, and encouraging them to follow the economic leadership of international institutions dominated by capitalist states. (p. 2)

The gradual introduction of social indicators was a shift in consciousness that marked a transition in international population and community development studies, which started contesting dominant knowledge systems and conventional economic measures as the main drivers of economic development (Haque, 2004). There was recognition that other important social and cultural aspects of progress and quality of life were as important for understanding economic growth and sustainable development (Helliwell, 2001; Helliwell & McKitrick, 1999; OECD, 2000).

The 1980s was also a significant time in the field of well-being as social and cultural indictors of well-being started to receive international attention. After the Brundtland Commission report of the late

1980s, it was generally accepted that the well-being of individuals and communities could not be defined and represented solely by economic growth and measures of GDP but needed to incorporate social, economic, and environmental dimensions (Brundtland Commission, 1987). Each of these dimensions has been defined in various ways by different interested parties ranging from the local scale to the international scale. For example, the World Health Organization's definitions of health suggest a holistic interpretation linking the complex inter-relationships among social, spiritual, economic, political, and cultural health determinants with the natural environment. This more comprehensive definition seems to be the one re-adopted for use by many Indigenous communities to develop their own tools for measuring well-being as demonstrated with FNPOW because it is more in keeping with their own holistic views (Cooke, 2005; Cooke et al., 2007; FNHA 2016d; White et al., 2009).

In 1990, the United Nations Development Programme made a major contribution to the development of composite indicators with the publication of the first Human Development Report. This report contained a new indicator, the HDI, which captured three dimensions of the development process – income, health, and knowledge – in a single indicator (Cooke et al., 2004; UNDP, 1990). The United Nations Development Programme has since refined some of these measures. For example, the HDI now "measures the average achievements in a country in three basic dimensions of human development: a long and healthy life, access to knowledge and a decent standard of living" (UNDP, 2016, n.p.) in its annual reports and has developed supplementary measures such as the Gender Inequality Index, which "reflects women's disadvantage in three dimensions – reproductive health, empowerment and the labour market" (UNDP, 2016, n.p.) and the Multidimensional Poverty Index, which "identifies multiple deprivations at the individual level in health, education and standard of living" (UNDP, 2016, n.p.).

The UNDRIP focuses on measures related to Indigenous health and well-being. For example, Article 21 states that:

1. Indigenous peoples have the right, without discrimination, to the improvement of their economic and social conditions, including, inter alia, in the areas of education, employment, vocational training and retraining, housing, sanitation, health and social security. 2. States shall take effective measures and, where appropriate, special measures to ensure continuing improvement of their economic and social conditions. Particular attention shall be paid to the rights and special needs of Indigenous elders, women, youth, children and persons with disabilities. (United Nations, 2008, p. 9)

And again in Article 24 there is particular attention to Indigenous tradition medicines and practices in relation to health whereby:

> Indigenous peoples have the right to their traditional medicines and to maintain their health practices, including the conservation of their vital medicinal plants, animals and minerals. Indigenous individuals also have the right to access, without any discrimination, to all social and health services. 2. Indigenous individuals have an equal right to the enjoyment of the highest attainable standard of physical and mental health. States shall take the necessary steps with a view to achieving progressively the full realization of this right. (UNDRIP, 2008, p. 9)

The United Nations Declaration on Rights of Indigenous Peoples serves as a critical step in addressing health inequalities experienced by Indigenous peoples across the globe and should be better integrated in measurement frameworks and indicators of health and well-being in Canada when we examine difference among Indigenous peoples and non-Indigenous peoples in Canada. According to Cooke (2005), "Canada's high ranking, including leading the list of countries with 'high human development' for most of the 1990s, became a point of pride for some Canadian politicians, despite the fact that there is very little difference in the Human Development Index scores of the most developed countries" (Cooke, 2005, p. 2). Moreover, it has been recognized that this high ranking in human development has not been experienced by Indigenous peoples in Canada (Cooke, 2005; Cooke et al., 2004).

On the contrary to what is happening, or more specifically what is *not* happening on a national level in Canada, the Happy Planet Index provides a measurement focus on human well-being in addition to rates of resource consumption. The New Economics Foundation, a registered charity founded in 1986 by the leaders of The Other Economic Summit, launched the Happy Planet Index in 2006:

> [The Index] identified health and a positive experience of life as universal human goals, and the natural resources that our human systems depend upon as fundamental inputs. This index has been regarded as an international measure that links human well-being to the environment with an underlying philosophy endorsing the premise that healthy societies are those that can support good lives and does not cost the Earth. (Daly, 2009, p. 3)

We also have much to learn in terms of measuring and assessing human well-being from Bhutan. In 2008, the Centre for Bhutan Studies launched the Gross National Happiness campaign to support a sustainability framework rooted in Buddhist philosophy and practice and a holistic approach to sustainable development. In addition to the conventional GDP figure, Bhutan also developed a Gross National Happiness Index comprised of nine dimensions: living standard, community vitality, culture, health, psychological well-being, education, environmental diversity, time use, and governance (Centre for Bhutan Studies, 2008). In Bhutan, the Gross National Happiness Index is used as the primary way to measure, evaluate, and track progress over time.

Other countries have focused on refining well-being frameworks and developing indicators linking human well-being to the environment. For example, the Australian Bureau of Statistics (2016) released the first ever Measures of Australia's Progress in 2002, which includes various social, economic, and environmental indicators aimed at tracking and measuring the country's progress. There are many social indicators ranging from health, education, and training to work, governance, and citizenship. Economic indicators have also been expanded to incorporate diverse forms of financial capital such as national income and wealth, household economic well-being, and housing conditions. The Measures of Australia's Progress also account for environmental indicators such as biodiversity, land, inland waters, oceans and estuaries, atmosphere, and waste (Australian Bureau of Statistics, 2016). In 2008, France put forward a key message emerging from the Commission on the Measurement of Economic Performance and Social Progress, stating that there is a need to "shift emphasis from a 'production-oriented' measurement system to one focused on the well-being of current and future generations, i.e., toward broader measures of social progress" (Stiglitz et al., 2010, p. 10). Hence, well-being is a multidimensional concept, and economic, social, cultural, and environmental dimensions should be considered simultaneously so that "quality-of-life indicators in all the dimensions covered should assess inequalities in a comprehensive way" (Stiglitz et al., 2010, p. 15).

There was also in the 1980s a shift in sociological thinking and a critique of socio-economic status as a measure of social status. For example, Goldman and Tickameyer's (1984) classic article on status attainment and human capital models sheds light on the extent to which, while describing the status of class relations in advanced capitalist systems, the models "ignore the historical roots and complex relations of uneven development between sectors" (Goldman & Tickameyer, 1984. p. 196), which in turn minimizes critical socio-historical context. This means that while status attainment models provide a measure of class relations categories in a hierarchical ordering of "minute gradients" (Goldman & Tickameyer, 1984, p. 207), at the same time the class relations categories reify stratification and class struggles by providing them with no historical context (Goldman & Tickameyer, 1984).

In addition, Blishen et al. (1987) present a Canadian socio-economic status index and at the same time critique the methodological tool as a social indicator based on the fact that such composite measures have enabled researchers to situate individuals within a complex, stratified division of labour. However, the "conceptual frameworks which have typically informed socioeconomic analyses theories of status attainment, of human capital, and of the functions of social stratification have met with increasing criticism from both Marxist and feminist scholars" (Blishen et al., 1987, p. 471) because the frameworks obscure relationships between gender and income. For example, Blishen et al. (1987) state that "even though their incomes may be highly disparate, women and men in identical occupations are by definition equal in their socioeconomic status" (Blishen et al., 1987, p. 477). In fact, the authors argue that despite the large gap between the median income of women ($7,847) and men ($15,804) in 1981, the median socio-economic score for women in the Canadian labour force is only slightly lower than the median score for men (Blishen et al., 1987). This article presents a socio-economic index for the total Canadian labour force based on 1981 Census data and clearly outlines the problems and criticisms of indexes of this kind. The authors suggest that the index is most applicable in circumstances where access to data is limited to occupational titles and where one desires a simple indicator that locates individuals in the Canadian occupational structure at a given point in time – otherwise, the index is problematic (Blishen et al., 1987).

How Is Well-being Measured in Canada?

In 2010, Human Resources and Skills Development Canada developed a group of indicators to measure well-being that examines the extent to which "individual Canadians and their families interact with each other and with social institutions over the course of their lives" (Foster & Keller, 2011, p. 10). This measurement tool incorporates a number of social and economic indicators expressed as resources and forms of social and economic capital. Interestingly, individuals and their families can build up and expend resources of different kinds (such as time, finances, goods and services, and social networks). Resources can be personal assets such as health and skills. Resources can also be the goods and services provided by social institutions. Finally, resources can be societal assets such as the environment and social order (Foster & Keller, 2011). The key social and economic domains embedded in this model include learning, "financial security, environment, security, health, leisure, social participation, family life, housing, and work" (Foster & Keller, 2011, p. 10).

Two main methods of measuring Indigenous community well-being in Canada have been developed and are composite measures of social and economic well-being used at the national and community levels: the Community Well-being Index (CWB) and the Registered Indian Human Development Index. Both indexes are adaptations of the United Nations HDI and were developed by the Strategic Research and Analysis Directorate of Aboriginal Affairs and Northern Development Canada in collaboration with various researchers and Indigenous communities (O'Sullivan, 2006). These indicators generally attempt to combine several important dimensions of Indigenous well-being into a single measure (a composite score) that can then be compared between communities and over time. As Cooke (2005) points out, "Each indicator must balance a desire to include the theoretically important dimensions of Indigenous well-being with ease of calculation and the availability and comparability of the data" (p. 1).

Most of the published literature surrounding Indigenous well-being is related to the measurement tools developed by INAC on the socio-economic status of these communities. The aim of these measurement tools has been to assess the well-being of Indigenous communities in relation to other Canadian communities. Much of the available literature on this aspect of First Nations well-being in Canada reports on the development of these tools and their various applications (Brink & Zeesman, 1997; Cooke et al., 2004; McHardy & O'Sullivan, 2004; O'Sullivan, 2006; White, Beavon, et al., 2007; White & Maxim, 2007; White, Wingert, et al., 2007). As mentioned, a number of publications regarding data sources, methodology, and current uses of the HDI and CWB by INAC and other government departments such as Human Resource Development Canada and Health Canada are available through the INAC website. The authors of the CWB recognize that the index focuses mainly on "mainstream" socio-economic aspects of well-being and does not take into account the differences in values or cultures between Indigenous and non-Indigenous communities or other aspects such as physical or psychological health (McHardy & O'Sullivan, 2004). However, the lack of available data that would allow comparisons between Indigenous and non-Indigenous communities means that the CWB is limited in scope. It focuses on only the four dimensions of well-being that are derived from Census of Population data and therefore the CWB is not reflective of the values of Indigenous ways of understanding well-being or even of Indigenous data sources.

Various measurement tools and indicators have been developed to measure community well-being in non-Indigenous communities, such as the Community Index of Wellbeing designed at the University of Waterloo that regularly reports on the quality of life of Canadians. But, in Canada, the ways of measuring the well-being of Indigenous peoples are still being developed. Indigenous world views and concepts of well-being emphasize a holistic view of health and wellness, often articulated by a balance of physical, mental, emotional, and spiritual dimensions which, again, are not reflected in the CWB, HDI, or the Community Index of Wellbeing. Although these dimensions are not easy to assess, they can be represented using conventional measurement tools and analytical methods rooted in socio-economic approaches informed by empirical data and quantitative measures (Cooke, 2009; White, Beavon et al., 2007; White & Maxim, 2007; White, Wingert, et al., 2007). Developing culturally appropriate measurement tools and indicators, which is the main focus of current research, has involved a collaborative effort between Indigenous organizations and government agencies. Through a cooperative knowledge approach, significant work has been completed in addressing both the issue of collecting reliable and comprehensive data and developing new ways of analysing the data such as the Regional Health Survey and the First Nations Regional Early Childhood, Education and Employment Survey. Given the diversity of Indigenous communities, many different approaches have been developed to assess the well-being of Indigenous individuals and communities, combining qualitative and quantitative research methods through an integrative research approach (Cooke. 2009; White, Beavon, et al., 2007; White & Maxim, 2007; White, Wingert, et al., 2007). Today, the most culturally relevant and up-to-date approach to conceptualizing the well-being of Indigenous communities is the FNPOW put forward by the FNHA in British Columbia. But there have been no substantial empirical efforts to implement and measure the dimensions within the perspective.

A review of the literature about well-being frameworks indicates there is no right way or perfect set of formulas for measuring wellness, while many recurring dimensions have been included in various frameworks (Helliwell, 2001). It is also important to note that, while some frameworks have begun to use the term "wellness," others have retained an overall health perspective yet include many subjective wellness indicators and prefer the term "perspective," which is the case for the FNPOW, rather than "model." A recent study pertaining to

Antonovsky's salutogenic model focuses on the origins of health and supports health promotion. The model explores the factors that support and increase well-being rather than merely on the factors that prevent disease (Antonovsky, 1996; Eriksson & Lindstrom, 2008; Lindstrom & Eriksson, 2009). This is a good example of a strengths-based approach to well-being because the model makes the assumption that wellness, not illness, is the norm for people. Interestingly, the model accounts for factors that enable people to remain healthy through so-called generalized resistance resources factors (Antonovsky, 1996) such as intelligence, financial resources, social support, knowledge, and traditions. The second model component that enables people to remain healthy is the "sense of coherence" that examines the ways in which people manage stress and resist illness (Antonovsky, 1996; Lindstrom & Eriksson, 2009). Overall, salutogenesis is gaining increasing acceptance as a useful model for promoting health and wellness and addressing health inequities (Billings & Hassem, 2009; Lindstrom & Eriksson, 2009).

How Is Indigenous Well-being Measured in Canada?

There has been a plethora of research dedicated to social capital in the context of Indigenous Nations and communities that heightens our understanding regarding how socially cohesive communities create bonds of trusting relationships and support the process whereby individuals and institutions can participate in community development projects (Carli, 2012; Chataway, 2002; Côté, 2012; Hill & Cooke, 2014; Mignone & O'Neil, 2005a, 2005b; Newhouse & Fitzmaurice, 2012). When we apply a two-eyed way of seeing it becomes clear that the "good life" can be viewed as a form of "social capital" (Bourdieu, 1972) reflecting the network of institutions and organizations within a community to deliver programs and services and the capacity of citizens within a community to engage in the activities offered through these programs and services. Processes of capacity building eventually become larger forms of social capital derived from sites of resource at the community and individual levels and foster good living. While there is debate in the literature about how to conceptualize and measure social capital, there is consensus about regarding it as a network of relationships between individuals and the communities in which they live. This network can be seen as a resource (Mignone, 2003; Mignone & O'Neil, 2005b) and takes a variety of forms such as good health, access to information and technological infrastructure, the practice of traditional knowledge systems, and opportunities that focus on supporting goals at individual and community levels (Hill & Cooke, 2014). As previously stated, there has been extensive research dedicated to exploring the extent to which socially cohesive communities support bridging processes for expanding community development (Chataway, 2002; Hill & Cooke, 2014; Mignone, 2003, 2009; Mignone & O'Neil, 2005b).

Social capital has been well identified in the literature as an important resource for community capacity building and a way of fostering the good life or Mino-Biimaadiziwin in an urban context (Hill & Cooke, 2014, Newhouse & Fitzmaurice, 2012). The Government of Canada, through various programs and policies such as the Urban Aboriginal Strategy, has been fostering research to provide solutions to deal with the growing Indigenous diaspora and a continued focus on providing solutions to deal with the so-called Indian problem (Newhouse & McGuire-Adams, 2012) in urban centres. The deficiency-based Indian problem approach to policy means little if any attempt has been paid to a strengths-based approach of looking at the areas of wellness such as through the determinants of health and wellness that could assist the development of good public policy (Newhouse & McGuire-Adams, 2012). A good understanding of this comes from the work of Hill and Cooke (2014) in this regard:

> Despite academic disagreements about how social capital is best defined or measured, improving these networks and trust relationships has become a focus for various community development schemes, with the idea that communities with higher degrees of social capital are better able to undertake particular projects or initiatives that respond to community defined needs, including improving access to various services and economic development initiatives. (p. 421)

The BC Progress Board was established in 2001 to measure the province's well-being performance in several key areas, including economic growth, standard of living, employment, environmental quality, health measures, and social conditions (BC Progress Board, 2010). The objective of this initiative is to gauge the extent to which quality of life in British Columbia is improving and to help advise on strategies and policies that could enhance the province's economic and social well-being and how the Province of British Columbia is ranked on its well-being performances relative to other Canadian provinces and the United States (BC Progress Board, 2010).

Another recent initiative in British Columbia that takes a strengths-based approach to well-being is the newly developed FNPOW advocated by the FNHA. The FNHA began its work in *re*-conceptualizing the health and wellness of First Nations communities throughout British Columbia in 2013. It has worked with communities across the Province of British Columbia to revitalize traditional knowledge systems and situate wellness within spiritual, emotional, mental, and physical contexts (FNHA, 2012). The FNPOW is innovative and is linked to Canada's Regional Health Survey data for selected reserve communities in British Columbia but can be used with other Indigenous data sources. The strength of the FNPOW is that it, unlike other ways of tracking and measuring wellness discussed to this point, is the first conceptual framework that has been designed from the grassroots. By this I mean that the dimensions used to create the FNPOW are based in Indigenous knowledge systems and incorporate holistic and natural medicines and innovative traditional and contemporary healing from an Indigenous perspective that are rooted in Indigenous values (FNHA, 2016d). The FNPOW supports a community strengths-based approach to wellness that moves from a sickness system of only looking at illness such as chronic disease to a wellness system that explores cultural and land-based practices and Indigenous languages. The wellness perspective also reflects that respect, responsibility and relationships, land, community, family and Nations, and social, environmental, cultural, and economic factors contribute to health and well-being (FNHA, 2011, 2016c).

Indigenous Health Indicator Frameworks

The 2012 Indigenous Health Indicator Frameworks were developed as an internal report for the Tripartite Health Indicators Planning Committee with the intention of examining existing frameworks – both Indigenous health indicator frameworks and frameworks with an awareness of Canadian Indigenous issues – to guide the Tripartite Health Indicator Planning Committee in creating a Health Indicator Framework for the FNHA (Laliberte, 2012). The report included a review of projects and identification of major themes in the international wellness literature. Laliberte (2012) suggests equity is a key component such that:

> Equity as an overarching dimension of a health indicator framework works well with an Indigenous health that works well with a "closing the gap" health agenda. (p. 6)

This requires a matching of key performance indicators between populations in order to capture measures to ensure that objectives are being met. Most of the projects, whether they were regional/national or community projects, used a systematic method of criteria-based indicator selection. "The Type of criteria, western and/or Indigenous, overlapped between projects and were formulated based on the conceptual 'place' of the organization, government department, or community" (Laliberte, 2012, p. 50).

Laliberte (2012) continues to argue that an important feature of the report is that, since it was prepapred by the FNHA, "the conceptual frameworks applied in Health Indicator Frameworks report 2012 reflect the values and beliefs of the people and organizations developing them" (p. 50). The author further emphasizes the importance of socio-cultural and wellness indicator domains as being "fundamental to community-based projects and are included in some of the regional/national Health Indicator Frameworks to a lesser degree" (Laliberte, 2012, p. 50). Self-determination and economic development have been identified in the Transformative Change Accord and tripartite agreements and are also themes in the First Nations Health Indicators Framework (Laliberte, 2012).

The FNPOW expands on the dimensions (mental, emotional, physical, and spiritual) depicted within the traditional Indian Medicine Wheel and represents a systematic form of knowledge that offers the potential to bridge Indigenous ways of knowing with the western knowledge system (FNHA, 2016d). In many Indigenous cultures, the Medicine Wheel metaphor contains traditional teachings and can be used as a guide for the re-introduction of Indigenous epistemologies into western knowledge systems, government policy, and academic discourse (Andreotti et al., 2011; Ashcroft, 2007; Beatty & Weber-Beeds, 2011; Berkman & Kawachi, 2000; Browne et al., 2005). While there is some variation in its teachings and representations, the underlying web of meaning in the Medicine Wheels remains the same: the importance of appreciating and respecting the ongoing interconnectedness and interrelatedness of all things (Ahenakew, 2011; Cajete, 2000).

Health and wellness are forms of social capital at the individual and community levels and many factors contribute to determining Indigenous health and wellness, for instance, past and current socio-economic status, affordable housing, employment, food security, safety, level of education, mental health, emotional wellness, and even a sense of Indigenous spirituality (Anaquot, 2006; Baum, 1998; Candland, 2000; Hill & Cooke, 2014). All of these factors have an impact on Indigenous peoples and their communities' health and well-being. As McCaslin and Boyer (2009) suggest:

> Decolonization helps communities resist factors that trigger crisis or place them at risk for future crisis. When crises or risk of crises arise, the response

must be framed by an understanding of the Indigenous context: the culture, the history, colonization, the nationhood of the people, and how their ways have been appropriated to serve the colonizing agenda. (p. 61)

A review of well-being frameworks and measurement tools reveals that the use of dimensions and indicators can be limited based on their conceptual design, the peoples for which they apply, and a lack of available and robust data sources. Indeed, the focus of this chapter has been to question how we understand knowledge, how this knowledge is generated, and, ultimately, how it is used. Colonization is ever present and deeply embedded in social structures such that "we are thoroughly acculturated to accept the colonial set-up as just the way it is ... education, social assistance, child welfare, and numerous other systems have installed colonial categories in our minds and inculcated colonial behaviours" (McCaslin & Boyer, 2009, p. 66).

It is crucial in the development of measurement frameworks and the selection of indicators that they reflect Indigenous knowledge systems; otherwise, we support and endorse colonial structures that continue to pathologize the health outcomes of Indigenous peoples, which is a step backwards along the pathway to reconciliation and self-determination. In Canada, colonization continues to provide the framework for enforcing the power relations that exist between Indigenous peoples and the rest of Canadian society. Laws, policies, and historical factors all affect the health and well-being of Indigenous peoples and how they have been implemented has added to a longstanding health gap for Indigenous peoples and communities. Research is an important step in reconciliation, but this step will be in the understanding and practice of the decolonization of research methodologies that will support the process of self-determination. This is really the starting point for what many scholars regard as the grounds for *real* conversations to occur about a renewed relationship between Indigenous peoples, the Canadian government, and non-Indigenous peoples (Blackstock, 2007; Corntassel, 2012; Denis, 2015; Simpson, 2011).

Central to many Indigenous cultures is the belief in the interconnectedness of all dimensions of one's life to the natural environment and this concept is widely expressed in the Indigenous community through the phrase "all my relations." This phrase implies that to live in harmony, one must balance all parts of life, including physical, mental, emotional, and spiritual well-being, within one's self, others, and the natural environment (Brave Heart, 1999a, 1999b). Well-being as conceptualized through the FNHA and, in particular, the FNPOW, is situated in Indigenous knowledge systems, reflects Indigenous knowledge systems, and is linked to the Traditional Medicine Wheel and ancestral teachings. Examining predictors of wellness through this lens enables researchers to identify health conditions and environmental factors such as culture, spirituality, behaviours, and adverse events that are associated with wellness. If moving forward in an era of reconciliation when new strategies and policies are to actually have a transformative effect on Indigenous peoples' lives, there must be a concerted effort to develop strategies that are community driven for change. Therefore, what is needed is seeking to understand the systemic structures of colonialism that operate in ways that are antithetical to Indigenous knowledge, teachings, and ways of life. This will create opportunities for decolonizing methodologies and strategies aimed at correcting power imbalances that have until now maintained the status quo.

5

Decolonizing Data and Critical
Research Methods

The chapter draws on the stories of thirteen key Indigenous participants using oral histories that are part of an FNHA case study. The knowledge created through these interviews traces the historical development of the FNPOW and, in doing so, describes a colonial continuum that reminds readers about the nature of knowledge creation and the extent to which knowledge is transformed into colonial practices that represent the interests of the powerful and serve to reinforce their positions in society with minimal benefit to fostering Mino-Bimaadiziwin or "the good life" among Indigenous peoples (Newhouse & Fitzmaurice, 2012). The conversation invites readers and users of this information to consider a different way to think about urban Indigenous health and well-being. In this chapter, I outline a research design based in a culturally respectful framework using mixed methodologies that does not place the value of western ways of understanding well-being over Indigenous ways of being well through the research process.

Through the example of my partnership with the FNHA, this chapter invites readers to consider the effectiveness of a research partnership that can braid useful western strands of research epistemologies with Indigenous forms of knowledge, world views, and cultural practices that are aligned with two-eyed seeing (Bartlett et al., 2012) to bridge differing world views between Indigenous and western knowledge systems. This chapter demonstrates how the FNPOW, developed through community engagement processes by the FNHA in British Columbia, offers an Indigenous way of looking at Indigenous health and wellness and serves to "decolonize bodies" by linking urban Indigenous wellness outcomes to traditional ancestral teachings and ways of being well that demonstrate Indigenous resistance and resilience (Strega & Brown, 2015) to ongoing structures of colonialism. This generates an important question for social researchers focusing on Indigenous issues: "How can western researchers work with Indigenous communities to better understand well-being?" This chapter presents findings that explore how engaging in traditional practices and cultural activities serves as the basis of well-being and how transgenerational trauma – most notably the impact of the residential school system – affects various aspects of well-being.

Decolonizing Methodologies

Academic institutions and researchers have a negative historical relationship with Indigenous peoples. Research practices are masked by scientific notions of objectivism rooted in a praxis of knowledge extraction from Indigenous communities in ways that serve to benefit the researchers and their institutions and advance disciplinary knowledge. These research processes reify existing power imbalances and reproduce colonial structures of western hegemonic discourses. Smith (2012) suggests that future research presented in an anticolonial framework must concentrate on both colonial relations and practice and create a critical link between theory and practice. In the end, the benefits of the research will be in creating a link through the culturally based knowledge interplay where Indigenous values, as they relate to well-being, are centralized at the onset of the research design process. This moves beyond theory to inform the ethics of practice in action-related research (Smith, 2012). The approach of this chapter supports the work of Indigenous resurgence scholars by showing that participation in Indigenous cultural activities is in and of itself an "act of everyday resurgence" (Corntassel, 2012; Hunt & Holmes, 2015) that serves to support Indigenous peoples to move towards building resilience and resources that have positive impacts on spiritual, physical, emotional, and mental wellness.

Indigenous scholars advocate that researchers engage in PAR because it is one of the methodologies that is acceptable when working with Indigenous communities (Castellano, 2004; Smith, 1999). The main reason for this preference is that the research design process of PAR studies reflects community-based research designs that incorporate a power-sharing process whereby the research benefits are shared by researchers and community. In addition, through PAR the actual research designs are more likely to be aligned with Indigenous world views that are rooted in a holistic tradition implicating health and well-being and that lead to action for change (Castellano, 2004; Corntassel 2012; Chester et al., 1994; Dickson, 2000; Fiske et al., 2001; Haig-Brown, 1992; Kenny, 2002; Simpson, 2011; Smith, 1999). Scholars have focused on the decolonization of social research methods by critically engaging with the dominant systems way of presenting research methods. This has been particularly evident in the works of Abolson (2011), Absolon and Willett (2005), Andersen and Walter (2014), Kovach (2005, 2009), Smith (1999, 2006, 2012), and Wilson (2008) by addressing issues of Indigenous relationality and ways of knowing and bringing forward an Indigenous research paradigm based in action.

Ethics: Honouring Indigenous Protocols and Relational Accountability

As a sociologist and community-based researcher, I regard the research work presented in this chapter as a way to bridge differences among Indigenous world views and non-Indigenous social research processes. The research presented here is supportive of Indigenous self-determination movements, especially the FNHA, and is a way to share my personal experiences and knowledge about the importance of the decolonization of research methods. Maintaining ethical standards is important and the research ethics boards at academic institutions, as well as individual researchers, still have some catching up to do when it comes to understanding Indigenous community protocols. The truth of the matter is that doing work with Indigenous peoples and community in research has less to do with university ethics–approved "engagement" research through stamps of approval and much more to do with genuine partnerships with agreed-upon ways of how knowledge is generated and shared within Indigenous knowledge networks and outside of these networks. This involves co-creating research design practices and ethical frameworks that are anchored in Indigenous ways of knowing. It requires understanding the principles of ownership, control, access, and possession (OCAP) as first introduced by the FNIGC and incorporating these principles into the early stages of a research design at the onset of a study. It requires that a person witness themselves as a researcher in the research process and ponder reflective questions about research transparency in the context of positionality, intentionality, power relationships, and accountability: "Who are you?" "Why are you here?" "What is the direct benefit of your research to the community?" (Absolon, 2011; Absolon & Willett, 2005; Kovach, 2005, 2009; Simpson, 2011; Smith, 1999). These questions are important and form the basis of the ethical manner in which I have carried out the research work. As researchers, I believe that we make choices about the work we do and how we intend to share our research with academic and non-academic audiences. This is an important aspect of addressing power relationships in research endeavours and why I decided to partner with the FNHA.

While I conducted my research in compliance with the University of Victoria Ethical Review Board, I also received permission from the FNHA Ethical Review Board and from every participant to conduct this research according to terms and conditions outlined in the Collaborative Research Agreement. Working exclusively within the parameters of university-approved ethical boards is incomplete. Such approaches to research are problematic especially when we consider that these practices reflect colonial ways of legitimizing research processes and reflect doing research "on" Indigenous peoples and communities as opposed to doing research "with" Indigenous peoples and communities. If we are to move forward in community-based scholarship, I believe that both types of reviews are crucial for transparent and meaningful research partnerships to occur; perhaps implementing a process that synthesizes these ethical review frameworks through a shared memorandum of understanding may be an area to explore in subsequent studies.

Participatory Action Research and Indigenous Communities

Participatory action research differs from most other approaches to Indigenous health and wellness research because it is based on reflection, knowledge co-creation, and action that aim to improve health and reduce health inequities through involving the people who, in turn, take actions to improve their own health (Castellano, 2004; Smith, 1999). The use of case study research is one of the main qualitative research traditions and falls under the umbrella of participatory action methods. The researchers' interest in the case may be *intrinsic* (the case drives the research) or *instrumental* (the case provides wider explanations and/or builds theories).[1] In both instances, a key virtue of case study methodology is its *holistic* approach to inquiry which, through data collection, incorporates multiple sources of information with the goal of generating in-depth knowledge processes (Stake, 2005; Verschuren, 2003; Yin, 2003, 2014). As a research strategy, a case study explores

---

1 While all qualitative case research should aim to provide an in-depth picture of that which is under study and pay close attention to context in all its detailed differentiation, a commitment to provide wider causal explanations through a case or to locate a case within a theoretical "set" can lead researchers to focus more closely on selected essential features of the case (Olsen, 2012).

a social issue or phenomenon "within its real-life context, especially when the boundaries between phenomenon and context are not clearly evident" (Yin, 2003, p. 13).

Two-eyed Seeing and Indigenous Health Outcomes

The qualitative data garnered through the study of First Nations health outcomes that I carried out in partnership with the FNHA can provide a knowledge basis supportive of a decolonized research process that bridges Indigenous world views with dominant knowledge structures. This type of research work is in line with what Mi'kmaw Elder of the Eskasoni First Nation, Alberta Marshall, has referred to as two-eyed seeing. Two-eyed seeing is using one eye to see health and wellness through Indigenous knowledge systems, and then using the other eye to see health and wellness through western-based knowledge systems. Using both knowledge systems is then combined to form two-eyed seeing, which will be beneficial to providing a more holistic lens to understanding health and wellness (Iwama et al., 2009). Further, this approach provides a bridging process and is an important contribution of this study because it is an initial stage in what Smith describes as the "decolonization of research methodologies" (Smith, 2012) and offers an approach to creating a space where traditional Indigenous knowledge and western discourse can be integrated into a shared knowledge system. This shared knowledge system will emerge in the creation of a conceptual framework and of wellness outcomes that can be used to better inform program and service delivery at the FNHA to enhance the lives of urban Indigenous peoples and communities.

In conversations with my research partner, the FNHA, we agreed that a case study framework would be most suitable for working with members of the FNHA in a way that did not obscure Indigenous knowledge and at the same time acted to bridge Indigenous and western knowledge systems. Specifically, the case study method was chosen due to its holistic approach and its conversational abilities, which are important considering that most First Nations teachings are delivered orally. In addition, I was invited to attend a one-day workshop on wellness indicators conducted on the Musqueam Indian reserve with (n=44) attendees who included staff from the FNHA and also community members; there were storytelling and knowledge sharing practices that helped to facilitate further knowledge acquisition for the case study through participant observation and memo taking.

In working in partnership with the FNHA, participants were selected from a public staff directory of key FNHA wellness staff members.

I selected participants based on a snowball sampling approach to conduct semi-structured personal interviews with FNHA staff in British Columbia that commenced in January 2016. This study used an oral history approach to data production so that rather than beginning with a hypothesis, the first step was collecting data through semi-structured telephone interviews; seven questions were used to keep the conversation focused on the FNPOW but were flexible enough to hold space for storytelling.

Qualitative Findings

One of my conversations with an Elder and Healer revolved around the topic of the FNPOW as a strengths-based approach to health and well-being. Part of the rationale provided as to why the FNPOW is regarded this way by Indigenous community members is based in Indigenous pedagogy and the concept of "all my relations." It is commonly understood among Indigenous peoples in Canada that interconnection is a central core of Indigenous world views and ways of knowing. This mindset reflects people who are aware that everything in the universe is connected. It also reinforces that everyone and everything has a purpose and a place in the grand scheme of life. First Nations relationships fully embrace the notion that people and their families are strongly connected to the communities they live in, their ancestors and future descendants, the land they live on, and all of the plants, animals, and other creatures that live upon it (Brave Heart, 2004; Cajete, 2004). During the conversation, the traditional Healer and Elder commented:

> Life is spiritual. The work we all did on the FNPOW was a spiritual journey. We are healers and it carries a spiritual energy. It's the farthest thing from western science. The perspective has its own life force. It is strength.

Several themes emerged from the conversations with key informants. The themes were analysed and then organized to create sets of subthemes. Each of the main themes and the subthemes provides valuable information and insight into all the interconnected knowledge systems that have been infused into the development of FNPOW, of its perceived benefits to the health and wellness of First Nations in British Columbia (individuals and communities), and of the depth of Indigenous knowledge that the perspective contains. The themes and subthemes are distinct and address relevant issues that cannot be omitted from a First Nations perspective on health and wellness. At the same time the themes and subthemes are interconnected, forming a wider picture. A working group within the FNHA was established to bring together a group of these knowledge holders who were in the best position to help support the FNPOW development process. Tradition is a core value and is reflected within the core values as the centre of FNPOW development. Traditional teachings and healing can only take place in community engagement. Community engagement efforts were regular and ongoing for all aspect of FNHA programming.

The Origin Story of the First Nations Perspective on Health and Wellness

The first question I asked of participants was "Why was the FNPOW created?" Three themes and two subthemes emerged. The first theme was to raise awareness and understanding by First Nations and the medical health system that BC First Nations do health differently. For change to occur, First Nations had to begin an exercise of articulating the difference: what do First Nations mean by "different" and how is "different" designed and implemented to improve health and close the gap between First Nations people and other people in Canada? To bridge the gap in knowledge is the next subtheme. Bridging the knowledge gap again requires articulation of First Nations knowledge and a comparison of the differences between that knowledge framework and western medical knowledge.

Commonality is about connection, unity, a shared discourse, and way of knowing and being in the world that comes from ancestral teachings and traditional knowledge systems. Commonality in interpretations of health and wellness is important when we consider that the FNPOW represents a diverse group of people (British Columbia has 200 First Nations Bands) with a shared history of colonization, intergenerational trauma, illness, and present-day shared priorities and interests of self-determination who are all walking the same journey towards wellness (FNHA, 2012b; Loppie-Reading & Wien, 2009; Reading et al., 2007). A movement away from a western model of illness and deficit-focused health system to a positive, strengths-based focus on wellness is a commonality and a resounding point of interest. A shift in thinking to a health and wellness orientation means that health-care service delivery and programming can broaden its scope to include an essence of spirituality that seriously questions possibilities within health prevention, health promotion, and traditional Indigenous healing. This broadening of perspective reflects First Nation values and is embedded in the FNPOW. It is not just another model to measure health outcomes per se; it is a way of relating to the social world and it is a way of life grounded in Indigenous knowledge. It can be applied in all areas of social life from policy development to boardroom conversations about best practices in community nursing and is supportive of two-eyed seeing.

Traditional Knowledge

The next theme explored "how" the model was created. For example, what knowledge and ideas were brought to the discussions and what knowledge informed these processes that gave the FNPOW its shape and form? Key informants explained that the participants looked to their traditional knowledge systems by way of ancestral teachings and storytelling for answers to the FNPOW design. They brought forth recollections, experiences, and wisdoms they were taught at home by parents and in the community by Elders. Traditional knowledge systems that included traditional teachings, traditional healing, and traditional wellness were all conceptions of tradition that informed that discussions.

Data Governance and Ownership

Data governance and ownership is an important theme related to the FNPOW and the responses to the question "Who does the FNPOW belong to – meaning who owns the FNPOW?" during the interviews were diverse. The question seemed to come full circle to a shared understanding that no one person or group could possibly own the FNPOW; everyone owns it. The FNPOW is linked to Indigenous peoples in communities and reflects community values and traditions that are rooted in ancestral teachings. While ownership is shared among people, it means that the medical profession and researchers, whether they are Indigenous or non-Indigenous, can benefit from the knowledge of the perspective but should apply the FNPOW in a respectful manner and ensure that when it is used it is with the intention of benefiting Indigenous peoples. The reason for this is that the FNPOW is a product of engagement of many representatives of First Nations people in British Columbia and the perspective can be applied to other Indigenous groups and would also well serve the non-Indigenous community.

From Illness Models to Wellness Perspectives

Figure 2 and figure 3 are examples of figures that are used to demonstrate the change in the community wellness scores from 1981 to 2011 for First Nations and Inuit and non-Indigenous communities in

Figure 2. Average community well-being index scores, First Nations and non-Aboriginal communities, 1981–2011

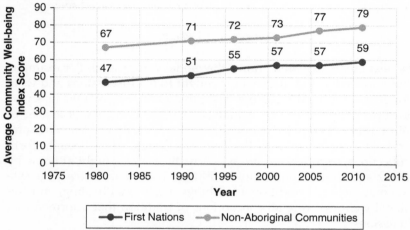

Source: INAC, 2015a; Statistics Canada, Censuses of Population, 1981–2006; and National Household Survey, 2011.

Canada. These scores are calculated by INAC and used to assess the "wellness" of Indigenous communities across Canada. In both cases, these visual displays of data show that the CWB gap between Indigenous peoples when compared to non-Indigenous peoples is substantial. INAC researchers calculated the 2011 CWB using data from the 2011 NHS. These data were made available to INAC and other external researchers in February 2014 through Statistics Canada's national network of Research Data Centres (INAC, 2015a).

From the results presented in figure 2 we can clearly see that the average CWB scores for First Nations communities are 20 percentage points below those for non-Aboriginal communities and this trend has been consistent, according to this measure, for three decades (1981–2011).

According to INAC, the CWB is used to assist its users to understand, track, and measure changes in well-being for Indigenous and non-Indigenous communities over time. In figure 3, from largest to smallest, the component gaps between First Nations and non-Aboriginal communities were as follows in 2011: income (25 points), education (17 points), housing (23 points), and labour force activity (16 points) (INAC, 2015a).

The data presented in figure 3 show the gap in CWB scores between First Nations and non-Aboriginal communities for each of the four main

Figure 3. Community well-being index component scores, First Nations and non-Aboriginal communities, 2011

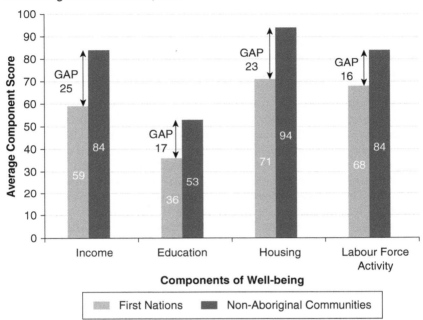

Source: INAC, 2015a; Statistics Canada, Censuses of Population, 1981–2006; and National Household Survey, 2011.

indicators used in the CWB calculation: income, education, housing, and labour force activity. This figure represents another way of highlighting a deficit approach to well-being for Indigenous communities.

As discussed in chapter 1, the CWB remains widely supported by federal government departments and continues to dominate the policy arena in Canada. It is clear from the above figures that there is a focus on well-being measurement and that by relying on four indicators (income, education, housing, and labour force activity) the CWB leaves out strength and wellness indicators. In doing so, it fails to tell a holistic story of health and wellness regarding Indigenous peoples. But a more pertinent question is what does a low CWB index score *mean*? Does the low value assigned to a community then serve to empower Indigenous peoples or the community in which they live? Obviously, the answer to this question is no. The FNHA identified a clear need for indicators that portray community strengths and resiliencies; this came in the form of feedback from the over 600 delegates who attended

the 2012 Gathering Wisdom V conference (FNHA, 2012). The dialogue
process among community members, Nations, leadership, and FNHA
staff has made the FNPOW instrumental in the development of a new
health and wellness model that will inform values, philosophies, and
cultures of First Nations communities across British Columbia (FNHA,
2012). The FNPOW is intended to aid in transformation of policy and
programming and in designs of innovative approaches to health and
wellness for First Nations across British Columbia. The FNPOW looks
at understanding health from a BC First Nations perspective, taking
into consideration regional variations in values, philosophies, and traditions. Included in this analysis is an interpretation of health as holistic, incorporating spiritual, emotional, mental, and physical domains, a
reflection of the Traditional Medicine Wheel (FNHA, 2016d). FNHA is
already using the model to move away from illness to a wellness system
of health. The perspective reflects Indigenous values from basic teachings that include respect, responsibility, and relationship to the land,
community, family, Nations, and social, environmental, cultural, political, and economic environments. This perspective is displayed visually
in figure 4 and has been developed through the history of health-care
provisions in British Columbia and the new tripartite arrangement of
the FNHA as previously discussed.

Figure 4 is the FNPOW, which has been derived from a holistic perspective and from the Medicine Wheel, which is based in four dimensions of health and wellness: spiritual, emotional, mental, and physical.
The people in the outer circle represent the vision of strong children,
families, Elders, and people in communities. The colours of the sunset
were chosen specifically to reflect the whole spectrum of sunlight and
to depict the sun's rotation around the earth, which governs the cycles
of life (FNHA, 2013b; FNHA 2016d). The basis of the FNPOW perspective is to evaluate health and wellness based on traditional knowledge,
ancestral teachings, and the understanding that all of these circles are
interconnected. Although the FNPOW appears in layers, it is important
to acknowledge that all the words in each circle are interconnected with
one other and with the components of other circles. For example, we
could regard the outer circle (environmental) to be linked to the next
circle (family) and the next circle (wisdom) and the next one (spiritual).
According to the interview participants, all the circles themselves are
interconnected and relate to each other. Ultimately, all of the factors
presented in the FNPOW are important and need constant rebalancing
in order to achieve wellness. It is critically important that there is balance among these dimensions of wellness and that they are all nurtured
in tandem to create a holistic level of well-being, one in which all four

Figure 4. First Nation perspective on wellness

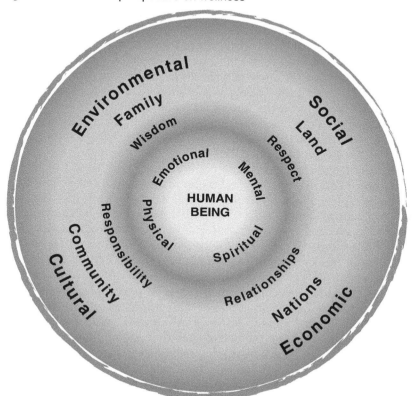

Source: FNHA, 2013b. Note that in more recent renditions the outside ring is accompanied by poeple holding hands.

areas are strong and healthy (FNHA, 2011, 2016d). Balance means that there are indicators for each of the four wellness dimensions: spiritual, emotional, physical, and emotional.

A Critical Data Approach

In a Foucauldian sense, social statistics have been used for state-building, as a mechanism for "governmentality," and as tools of social control for the population and the site at which political power operates (Foucault, 1972). The way in which Indigenous peoples have encountered social statistics by the Canadian government is linked to the residential school system when each student's Indigenous name was removed and replaced by a number. For example, the TRC's report (2015) points out that it was common practice that the moment Indigenous children entered residential schools, their identities were stripped when their Aboriginal names were replaced with Euro-Canadian ones and each student was assigned a number (Sellars, 2013). Teachers would often refer to students only by their numbers (TRC, 2015). These sorts of practices are rooted in settler state–Indigenous relations and so the use of social statistics continues to raise concerns about who benefits from applied research and how social statistics are used when working with Indigenous peoples and communities (Andersen & Walter, 2014).

Critical theorists suggest that what is needed is to "seek a sociology that is grounded in empirical and theoretical research *and* that hones a critical perspective less restricted by established institutions" (Feagin, 2004 in Carroll, 2004, p. 37). This will in turn "alert us to the need for critical researchers employing quantitative methods to do so in ways that are broadly consonant with the ontological and ethical commitments of the social analysis" (Carroll, 2004, p. 390). In their book *Indigenous Statistics: A Quantitative Research Guide*, Andersen and Walter (2014) provide a critical look at the ways in which quantitative data has restricted our understanding of Indigenous peoples and Indigenous issues. Andersen and Walter (2014) are clear in making a strong case for the fact that the methodologies that are applied to produce statistics include the ways research questions are asked; how the data are collected, analysed, and reported are not neutral or mere "descriptions" of artefacts. Statistics come with underlying values and methodologies that reflect and constitute the dominant cultural framework and not the values of Indigenous world views. This has caused harm to many Indigenous peoples in "creating a public understanding of Indigenous peoples in terms of deficit and dysfunction and the problem in society" (Andersen & Walter, 2014, p. 10). Critical theorists and Indigenous scholars recognize that population statistics, and quantitative research methods more generally, are rooted in a positivist tradition (Apparurai, 1993). The FNPOW has been developed through a localized knowledge process and it is imperative to understand this development process from the standpoint of the FNHA because it is reflective of traditional knowledge systems and integral aspects of the well-being of urban Indigenous peoples based on a more holistic perspective of well-being. This is a culturally responsive and decolonized approach to understanding well-being in both the framework and in the use of the survey data and analysis provided in the following sections.

Decolonizing Data and Indigenous
Health Outcomes

By applying the FNPOW, the quantitative component of this chapter examines the general attributes and indicators (specific measurable items) that can be drawn from data to empirically assess the determinants of health and wellness for the Indigenous diaspora. The 2012 APS is Canada's national survey of First Nations, Métis, and Inuit people living in urban centres across Canada.[2] The APS has been conducted by Statistics Canada since 1991 and the data generated from this survey provide a range of socio-economic and health and wellness indicators about Indigenous peoples in Canada. The 2012 APS was drawn from a sample of more than 50,000 respondents who identified as "Aboriginal" in the 2011 NHS and of this sample approximately 38,150 individuals completed the survey for a total response rate of 76%. Excluding the 9,740 non-Aboriginal respondents, the total number of Indigenous respondents in the APS is 28,410 (Statistics Canada, 2012).[3]

The 2012 Aboriginal Peoples Survey
and Measuring Historical Trauma

For the multilevel analysis, the multilevel structure operationalized for the analysis from the 2011 NHS consists of $n = 1,111,860$ Indigenous individuals nested within 147 communities comprised of both CMAs and CAs.[4] However, the total population size of the First Nations com-

2 The content for the 2012 APS was developed by Statistics Canada in collaboration with the three federal funding departments: INAC (formerly called Aboriginal Affairs and Northern Development Canada), Health Canada, and Employment and Social Development Canada (formerly called Human Resources and Skills Development Canada). In addition, the framework guiding content development also was developed during engagement and consultation sessions with the Canadian Council on Learning in partnership with First Nations, Inuit, and Métis communities and organizations across Canada (Cloutier & Langlet, 2014).
3 The study included all First Nations peoples 20 years of age and older living in CMA (population size >100,000) and CA (population size >10,000 but <100,000) urban communities across Canada. The 2012 APS did not ask any trauma-related questions of anyone under the age of 19 and so this group of people were not part of the present analysis. The inclusion criteria used for analysis were (1) all Indigenous peoples who identify as First Nations, (2) First Nations peoples aged 20 years and older since they were asked the residential school attendance question and other subsequent trauma-related questions, and (3) First Nations peoples living in non-rural areas.
4 For more information about census and geographic concepts, please see http://www.statcan.gc.ca/pub/93-600-x/2010000/definitions-eng.htm

munity is 366,166 peoples that self-identified as First Nations (only). According to Statistics Canada (2016), a CMA must have a total population of at least 100,000 of which 50,000 or more must live in the urban core. A CA must have an urban core population of at least 10,000.

The 2012 APS indicates that approximately 17% of First Nations peoples live in CMAs (population > 100,000) and in CA areas (population > 10,000). The sample size used in this analysis is $n = 4,811$ First Nations peoples, the composition of the sample is 49.8 per cent male and 50.2 per cent female, and the mean age is 38.2 years (Statistics Canada, 2016). The results in table 1 show the average Transgenerational Trauma Index (tgtindex) score across 71 communities in Canada.[5] The communities with the highest levels of trauma are Yorkton, Saskatchewan; Lethbridge, Alberta; Brandon, Manitoba; Regina, Saskatchewan; and Port Alberni, British Columbia. It is important to note that these transgenerational trauma values are not proportional to population size. That is, as the number of First Nations peoples in a city increases, it does not mean that the average score of transgenerational trauma increases. For example, Yorkton, Saskatchewan has the highest level of transgenerational trauma when compared to other communities although the population of First Nations peoples in Yorkton is 870 people. Compare this to a larger urban centre such as Vancouver where there are 20,080 First Nations peoples and the transgenerational trauma value is much lower.

The impacts of residential schools are transgenerational; many Indigenous peoples are born into families and communities that have been struggling with the effects of trauma for many years. According to the First Nations Information Governance Centre (2012) in the 2008/2010 Regional Longitudinal Health Survey "A higher proportion of First Nations adults with a chronic health condition reported moderate to high levels of depression (34.4% vs. 20.8), [and] suicide ideation (24.3% vs. 17.7) ... compared to those without a chronic health conditions" (FNIGC, 2012, p. 118). These findings are useful and can be a guide to understanding the magnitude of transgenerational trauma especially in smaller communities where there may not be sufficient social programs and services to support First Nations peoples in dealing with the impacts of residential school trauma.

---

5 Statistics Canada suppression rules would not permit communities with cell counts less than 10 people in the unweighted result to be released for the 2012 APS confidential data file. The consequence is that the tgtindex value for 76 communities could not be included in the transgenerational trauma Table 7.

Table 1. Transgenerational trauma index by community

Community	First Nations Population	Average Index Score
Corner Brook	3,360	0.1
Halifax	3,820	0.3
Fredericton	1,200	1.1
Quebec	3,840	0.4
Montreal	11,590	0.6
Ottawa – Gatineau (Quebec part)	4,020	0.2
Ottawa – Gatineau (Ontario part)	7,200	0.9
Belleville	1,900	0.8
Peterborough	720	1.2
Oshawa	2,740	0.3
Toronto	19,220	0.7
Hamilton	5,030	0.7
St. Catharines – Niagara	5,210	0.4
Kitchener – Cambridge – Waterloo	3,210	0.5
Brantford	3,160	0.9
London	4,540	0.6
Chatham-Kent	1,140	0.7
Windsor	3,010	0.3
Sarnia	2,870	0.7
Barrie	840	0.5
Orillia	1,150	0.5
North Bay	2,130	0.9
Greater Sudbury	3,110	0.9
Timmins	900	1.0
Sault Ste. Marie	2,470	0.7
Thunder Bay	7,190	1.7
Kenora	830	1.0
Winnipeg	18,890	1.8
Portage la Prairie	890	**2.2**
Brandon	1,120	**2.9**
Thompson	2,590	1.4
Regina	6,420	**2.9**
Yorkton	870	**3.3**
Moose Jaw	150	2.3
Saskatoon	5,650	1.5
North Battleford	1,310	1.6
Prince Albert	5,610	2.2
Medicine Hat	1,200	0.7
Lethbridge	1,370	**3.2**
Calgary	8,330	1.8
Red Deer	1,420	2.2
Edmonton	16,430	1.6
Grande Prairie	1,480	2.1
Wood Buffalo	1,530	1.0
Cranbrook	380	1.8

(*Continued*)

Table 1. (Continued)

Community	First Nations Population	Average Index Score
Kelowna	2,130	0.9
Vernon	1,890	1.6
Kamloops	2,440	1.1
Chilliwack	3,560	1.8
Abbotsford – Mission	2,330	1.2
Vancouver	20,080	1.2
Victoria	5,240	**2.4**
Duncan	960	2.2
Nanaimo	2,780	1.4
Port Alberni	510	**2.7**
Courtenay	1,450	1.3
Campbell River	1,870	1.6
Williams Lake	1,290	2.0
Quesnel	820	1.4
Prince Rupert	2,570	1.6
Terrace	2,770	1.6
Prince George	2,940	1.9
Fort St. John	860	1.7
Whitehorse	2,100	2.2
Yellowknife	1,520	2.8

Source: 2012 Aboriginal Peoples Survey

Individual- and Community-level Factors Affecting Indigenous Health Outcomes

As discussed at the onset of this book, residential schools have created various forms of trauma that continue to affect the lives of Indigenous peoples – trauma directly affects individuals who attended residential schools and also affects different generations of family members who feel the effects of this trauma. However, the impacts of colonialism are not restricted to residential schools but extend to a number of social, cultural, and economic conditions that have negative effects on Indigenous peoples' sense of well-being. It is common knowledge among researchers that as individuals we live in communities. If the communities in which we live are experiencing high rates of trauma and other related social and cultural conditions then this could have strong impacts on the individuals who live in those communities. The focus of this section of the chapter is to examine the ways in which community-level factors affect individual levels of well-being for First Nations peoples living in urban centres across Canada.

A multilevel modelling approach supports researchers with looking at the relationships between socio-economic and cultural factors on individual health and wellness outcomes, and at the same time looking at how community factors influence individual health and wellness outcomes.[6] It is important to recognize that there are considerable variations in Indigenous health and well-being dimensions among Indigenous peoples. The determinants of health and wellness are best understood in a multivariate context that accounts for their interconnections and the combined effect they have on different aspects of individual and community-level health and well-being. Most statistical techniques assume that observations in the dataset are independent from each other but when groups of observations share some features in common, then they are no longer independent (Heck & Thomas, 2015) especially when these features are related to geographic proximity or network membership. When the data have information at different levels, such as at the individual level and at the community level, the data are said to be hierarchical (Heck & Thomas, 2015). Multilevel modelling analysis is a useful technique when we consider that individuals interact with their social contexts and that between-individual differences in individual attributes might either be affected by collective attributes as confounding variables and/or as contextual effects influencing the direction and/or magnitude of the individual-level effects, which in the terminology of the literature are called "cross-level interactions" (Heck & Thomas, 2015, p. 43).

Four dependent variables are modelled after the Traditional Medicine Wheel and used for analysis in this study: emotional wellness, physical wellness, mental wellness, and spiritual wellness. These are shown in figure 5.[7]

---

6 In the multilevel analysis, I created a separate data file using the 2011 NHS based on 146 communities. The preparatory step in the multilevel analysis was in creating a level 1 (individual) data file using the 2012 APS and also creating a level 2 (community) data file based on community estimates using the 2011 NHS. These two separate data files were merged to create one master data file and to estimate the community level effects on the four dimensions of Indigenous health and wellness (the Traditional Medicine Wheel) as discussed.

7 First, the variance of the intercepts was examined to determine whether each of the variances were different from zero. In all cases, except for the spiritual variable, the variances were significantly different from zero. These models became the "null models" against which other models were assessed (for example, for purposes of ascertaining level-2 R squares). Next, the Random Intercepts Models were expanded to include community-level independent variables. Random Slopes models are analogous to interaction models in regular regression modelling. They allow for the possibility that the effect of a level-1 variable might itself be contingent on some level-2 variable. For example, in the case of this study the effect of participation in arts and crafts might itself be contingent on community size.

Figure 5. The influence of multilevel model variables on the four dimensions of the Traditional Medicine Wheel

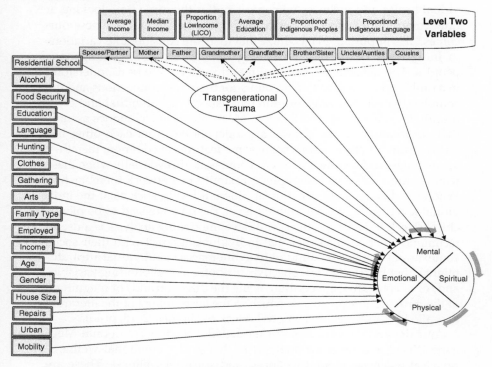

Source: Quinless, J. (2017). Decolonizing Bodies: A First Nations Perspective on the Determinants of Urban Indigenous Health and Wellness in Canada, p. 236. PHD Dissertation, University of Victoria.

Quantitative Findings

Table 2 presents the coefficients and table 3 shows the fitted values for different conditions for ease of interpretation (for the "arts" variable) and different levels for two significant community-level variables on physical wellness, which are the proportion of (1) First Nations peoples who speak an Indigenous language and (2) people living on an urban reserve. These results are important and show that there are higher levels of physical wellness in those communities where there is a higher proportion of First Nations peoples speaking an Indigenous language and living on an urban reserve. However, statistically speaking we also see what is called a crossover effect, which means that the effects of community variables are in the opposite direction and contingent on

Table 2. Results of multilevel random slopes – physical wellness (low score)

Information	Criteria			
	Akaike	(AIC)	13,835.691	
	Bayesian	(BIC)	14,014.694	
	Sample-Size	Adjusted BIC	13,925.722	

Level 1: Individual

		Estimate	S.E.	Est./S.E.	P-Value
	Gender	−0.181	0.064	−2.814	**0.005**
	Alcohol Consumption	−0.059	0.014	−4.22	**0.000**
	Transgenerational Trauma Index	0.016	0.026	0.629	0.529
	5-Year Mobility	0.014	0.022	0.616	0.538
	Highest Level of Schooling	−0.046	0.022	−2.102	**0.036**
	Indigenous Language Ability	−0.025	0.027	−0.917	0.359
	House Repairs Needed	0.140	0.053	2.659	**0.008**
	Indigenous Clothes/ Footwear	0.065	0.100	0.653	0.514
	Age	0.034	0.002	14.924	**0.000**
	Family Type	−0.154	0.063	−2.448	**0.014**
	Traditional Hunting/Fishing	0.066	0.055	1.198	0.231
	Traditional Gathering of Berries/Plants	0.093	0.065	1.427	0.153
	Household Size	−0.031	0.021	−1.513	0.130
	Employed	−0.303	0.065	−4.646	**0.000**
	Attended Residential School	−0.072	0.099	−0.725	0.469
	Urban	0.015	0.073	0.210	0.833
	Level of Food Security	−0.361	0.077	−4.683	**0.000**
	Income	0.002	0.006	0.306	0.760

Level 2: Community

Cross-Level Interactions	Indigenous Language × Arts	**−2.231**	0.671	−3.323	0.001
	Proportion on Reserve × Arts	**−0.428**	0.298	−1.437	0.151
	Intercepts				
	Physical Wellness	1.201	0.074	16.276	0.000
	Indigenous Arts/Crafts	0.349	0.112	3.13	0.002
	Indigenous Language	0.659	0.544	1.211	0.226
	Urban Reserve	−0.101	0.118	−0.852	0.394

Note: Bold indicates statistically significant results.

Table 3. Results of fitted values of multilevel random slopes – physical wellness

Arts by Language

| | Language | | |
	Low	Mean	High
Arts	0	0.05	0.02
Yes	1.673	1.559	1.218
No	1.612	1.549	1.360

Arts by Reserve

| | Reserve | | |
	Low	Mean	High
Arts	0	0.3	0.6
Yes	1.686	1.573	1.251
No	1.607	1.543	1.349

participating in arts/crafts. Generally, we see in this model that the proportion of First Nations who speak an Indigenous language and the proportion of people living on reserves is positive for the random slope of arts/crafts leading to higher physical wellness scores in communities with *low language use* among First Nations and in communities with a low proportion of people living on urban reserves. Interestingly, we also see that communities with *high language use* or a higher proportion of urban reserves leads to lower physical wellness scores. This finding is consistent with previous findings and reinforces the point that physical wellness is associated with participation in traditional cultural activities such as arts and crafts and also with language use.

The results also show that a number of individual socio-economic and cultural attributes continue to be significant in affecting physical wellness, including gender, housing in need of repairs, employment, and level of food security. Overall, this model tells us that males experience more physical wellness compared to females but this varies across urban communities. We also see that those living in houses in need of major repairs and in homes with low levels of food security, as well as those who are unemployed, also experience lower levels of physical wellness.

Table 4 presents the coefficient and table 5 presents the fitted values for ease of interpretation. This model looks at individual and community effects on emotional wellness. The results indicate that the proportion of First Nations peoples who speak an Indigenous language within a community affects emotional wellness. We also see that people with

Table 4. The predictors of the slope of arts – emotional wellness

Information	Criteria			
	Akaike	(AIC)	13,230.17	
	Bayesian	(BIC)	13,421.959	
	Sample Size	Adjusted BIC	13,326.631	

Level 1: Individual

	Estimate	S.E.	Est./S.E.	P-Value
Emotional Wellness	ON			
Alcohol Consumption	0.019	0.012	1.616	0.106
Attended Residential School	0.000	0.115	0.000	1.000
Level of Food Security	0.345	0.04	8.564	0.000
Traditional Gathering of Berries/Plants	0.096	0.056	1.707	0.088
Gender	−0.074	0.056	−1.315	0.189
5-Year Mobility	−0.034	0.016	−2.165	0.03
Highest Level of Schooling	0.054	0.025	2.203	0.028
Indigenous Language Ability	0.013	0.025	0.503	0.615
House Repairs Needed	-0.074	0.049	−1.521	0.128
Indigenous Clothes/ Footwear	0.048	0.085	0.566	0.571
Age	−0.004	0.002	−2.192	0.028
Family Type (second generation vs. multigeneration)	0.097	0.047	2.061	0.039
Traditional Hunting/Fishing	0.025	0.053	0.467	0.641
Household Size	0.008	0.02	0.412	0.680
Employed	0.007	0.048	0.146	0.884
Urban	−0.092	0.06	−1.546	0.122
Income	0.007	0.004	1.578	0.115
Residual	Variances			
Emotional Wellness	1.106	0.077	14.35	0.000

Level 2: Community

	Estimate	S.E.	Est./S.E.	P-Value
Arts × Indigenous Language	−1.016	0.516	−1.968	0.049
Tgtindex × Indigenous Language	−0.887	0.318	−2.791	0.005
Indigenous Language	−1.511	0.376	−4.023	0.000
Slope of Arts	−0.010	0.026	−0.391	0.696
Slope of Tgtindex	0.005	0.007	0.776	0.438
Intercepts				
Emotional Wellness	1.627	0.071	23.067	0.000
Arts	0.061	0.071	0.857	0.391
Tgtindex	0.079	0.026	3.077	0.002

Table 5. Results of fitted values of multilevel random slopes – emotional wellness

Arts by Language

	Language		
	Low	Mean	High
Arts	0	0.05	0.2
Yes	1.673	1.559	1.218
No	1.612	1.549	1.360

TgtIndex by Language

	Reserve		
	Low	Mean	High
Arts	0	0.3	0.6
Yes	1.686	1.573	1.251
No	1.607	1.543	1.349

transgenerational trauma have higher emotional wellness (support systems) and also that people participating in arts have higher levels of emotional wellness.

Transgenerational Trauma and Health Outcomes

The experience of high rates of trauma has an impact on all dimensions (spiritual, physical, mental, and emotional) of individual levels of well-being. At the community level, the results in table 5 show that trauma continues to be an important predictor of emotional wellness alongside participation in arts and crafts. This suggests that residential school attendance had results in negative experiences that are cumulative over time and culturally transmitted among family members. Transgenerational trauma leads to lower levels of spiritual, physical, mental, and emotional wellness among urban First Nations peoples across communities.

Indigenous Culture as Resistance to Trauma

Another important finding in this chapter is that there is strong empirical evidence that supports that participation in Indigenous arts and crafts and language use offsets some of the adverse impacts of colonialism. These cultural determinants of health and wellness serve as forms of resilience and provide traditional medicine that can be used to help close the health gap. These results are important because they reframe the determinants of health from socio-economic factors to an emphasis on the importance of addressing health inequalities by focusing on Indigenous cultural activities. The FNPOW is especially useful in studies of the determinants of health and wellness because it incorporates innovative practices such as holistic and natural medicines and spiritual and traditional knowledge from a First Nations perspective (FNHA, 2013). Understanding that colonialism is the seed of trauma that manifests itself through health and wellness leads to economic and political dependency (Alfred, 2009). This dependency is an Indigenous community's economic, social, and political structures being tied to colonial structures such as education outcomes and income (Alfred, 2009).

In summary, the FNPOW was developed as recently as the 1980s but the knowledge systems that are embedded within the perspective are rooted in a time of pre-settler contact (FNHA, 2016d). It is an organic and fluid way of seeing and relating to the world that incorporates evolving thoughts about the conception and operation of health and wellness among Indigenous peoples across British Columbia. Applying the FNPOW to Indigenous survey data provides the opportunity to generate decolonized health and wellness outcomes, a pathway to decolonizing bodies. This becomes apparent when we look at the national measurement of Indigenous well-being through the CWB and the way in which it continues to perpetuate a deficit approach to Indigenous health and wellness.

The main findings in this study point to a need for future quantitative research to consider the influence of health and wellness factors that reflect Indigenous knowledge systems and community values. In particular, the models presented in this chapter are useful when thinking about the determinants of health and wellness because they reveal the importance of comparing different dimensions of health and wellness that are further linked to different geographical areas and communities within the urban landscape across Canada. The results demonstrate that transgenerational trauma, residential school attendance, food security, alcohol use, and participation in Indigenous land-based traditions, language use, and cultural activities are significant in predicting a variety of wellness outcomes. The qualitative data generated in this study explain how the FNPOW is anchored in Indigenous traditional knowledge systems, community values, the self-determined strength of individuals, and the organizational capacity of the FNHA in British Columbia. The research then applies the FNPOW to the 2012 APS data and the 2011 NHS using quantitative analysis to generate indicators of health and wellness that are culturally relevant and more aligned with Indigenous world views.

6

Conclusion

Scholars have focused on the decolonization of qualitative and quantitative research methods by critically engaging with the dominant systems way of presenting research methods. This has been particularly evident in the works of Absolon (2011), Absolon and Willett (2005), Andersen and Walter (2014), Kovach (2005, 2009), Smith (1999, 2006, 2012), and Wilson (2008) that centre Indigenous ways of knowing and offer Indigenous research paradigms based on action. The approach of this book is different from other works in the field because it is written from the standpoint of a non-native scholar applying a decolonization approach to social scientific methods. My writing is not based in Indigenous methodologies or ceremonies per se but rather critically examines common social research methods from an insider perspective through a decolonizing standpoint that is a strengths-based approach to health and wellness research. A strengths-based approach to research involves a concerted effort to focus on what is working well within Indigenous communities as opposed to identifying and accentuating problems and deficits. The findings outlined in this book also support a two-eyed way of seeing health and wellness by showing that a strengths-based approach to well-being can be regarded as a form of social capital and that well-being can be a resource utilized by Indigenous peoples to invest in and experience wellness and strengthen their lives and local communities. This was explained through the research partnership with the FNHA and by applying the FNPOW. All of this was guided by Indigenous ethical frameworks and grounded in community ways of understanding health and well-being. The position I have taken in this book is that a critical research approach and decolonizing stance with respect to research data can be transformed to be culturally responsive. As well, PAR can be inclusive of multiple epistemologies (qualitative and quantitative research approaches) and traditional Indigenous knowledge systems in constructing a strengths-based perspective to understanding urban Indigenous well-being.

The findings of the study are used to illustrate a decolonizing approach to standard social science research methods widely supported in the field of sociology but the study is different in that it also supports the work of Indigenous health advocates. In terms of illustrating a decolonizing approach, the qualitative data generated through a case study approach using oral histories explains how the FNPOW is anchored in Indigenous traditional knowledge systems, community values, and the self-determined strength of individuals and the organizational capacity of the FNHA in British Columbia. In terms of supporting Indigenous health advocates, I applied the FNPOW to the 2012 APS data and the 2011 NHS data using a quantitative analytical strategy to generate indicators of health and wellness that are culturally relevant and more aligned with Indigenous world views according to the teachings of a two-eyed seeing perspective. The overarching findings provided a two-eyed way of seeing Indigenous health and wellness outcomes. In fact, the health and wellness outcomes revealed that participation in Indigenous cultural activities are in and of themselves an "act of everyday resurgence" (Corntassel, 2012; Corntassel & Scow, 2017; Hunt & Holmes, 2016) that serves to support Indigenous peoples to move towards building resilience and resources that have positive impacts on spiritual, physical, emotional, and mental wellness. These findings and the methods used to generate them invite readers and users of this information to consider an alternative way to think about urban Indigenous health and well-being.

Indigenous-based Determinants of Health and Wellness

The FNPOW is especially useful in studies of the determinants of health and wellness because it incorporates innovative practices such as holistic and natural medicines along with spiritual and emotional counsel from a First Nations' perspective, and practices that reconnect with the spirit, land, and communities. In a health and wellness–centred environment, it is possible to use and affirm existing Indigenous approaches to health, advocate and collaborate with partners to promote and invest in health and wellness, and support health promotion and disease prevention approaches in partnerships. The FNPOW also reflects that respect, responsibility and relationships, land, community, family and Nations, and social, environmental, cultural, and economic factors contribute to health and well-being, Understanding that colonialism is the seed of trauma, this book provides empirical support for the ongoing impacts of transgenerational trauma and the way it impacts different aspects of health and wellness.

In terms of policymaking, future research endeavours must continue to acknowledge and investigate the distinct influence of transgenerational trauma on Indigenous peoples' health and well-being. This acknowledgment should be supplemented with learning and understanding the ways the impacts of trauma are mediated through Indigenous resurgence of speaking Indigenous languages and participation in cultural activities such as arts and crafts, making traditional clothes and footwear, and land/water-based practices such as gathering medicines, berries, sweet grass, and so forth. Understanding current and transgenerational impacts on health and wellness holds important potential to guide policy and to redress the social, economic, and political context that lies at the root of urban health disparities for Indigenous peoples. In working towards enhancing the lives of Indigenous Nations, peoples, and communities, policymakers must consider the colonial context in which health is linked and the ways in which different dimensions of health and wellness are interconnected and experienced. There is still much work ahead in the nexus of social inequality, health disparities, social capital analysis, and understanding where these realities are situated in this colonial world. The decolonization of research methodologies has been a leading research priority for over two decades (Bishop, 2005; Smith, 2012) and is widely recognized as being emancipatory and inciting positive social change (Smith, 2006, 2012) within the international Indigenous community. It is time that researchers from all disciplines start doing research in different ways.

Social Capital and Indigenous Health and Wellness

As previously discussed, social capital analysis has been widely regarded as a particularly useful lens to understanding how ongoing colonial structures and polices serve to disenfranchise Indigenous communities' investments in health and wellness (Baum, 1998). From a Bourdieusian perspective, a more general understanding about how the CWB and other related measures of health and well-being for Indigenous peoples and communities come to represent categories of power that are continually invested in by those in positions of power. The scores generated from the CWB index reflect the knowledge systems and values based in western thinking, in which CWB normalizes Indigenous health and wellness according to non-Indigenous ways of knowing. Social capital analysis is also useful as Veenstra (2002) points out, whereby at the community level we can understand the importance of social capital as linkage that may affect population health by increasing accessibility to health services. He finds, "The inclusion of rural areas ... brings the relevance of income inequality as a predictor of a population's health back on stage in Canada" (Veenstra, 2002, p. 865) and this is what is needed in developing a common understanding and in developing responsive policies. Chandler and Lalonde (1998) have demonstrated that the ability of a group to develop linkage social capital is also implicated in the maintenance of cultural continuity, as evidenced in their work that examined the importance of cultural continuity in reducing suicidal ideation among First Nation youth. They found that cultural continuity is a main protective factor against suicide and "the communities that have taken active steps to preserve and rehabilitate their own cultures are also those communities in which youth suicide rates are dramatically lower" (Chandler & Lalonde, 1998, p. 18).

The findings presented in this book have demonstrated how understanding health and wellness from an Indigenous standpoint and applying the FNPOW to national level survey data such as the 2012 APS and the 2011 NHS produce determinants of health and wellness that are more meaningful to urban Indigenous peoples. But I think this is only a starting place and Indigenous data sources need to be expanded and support provided for Indigenous data initiatives outside of federal government jurisdiction that are community-driven. The findings of chapter 5 show that while all aspects of emotional, physical, mental, and spiritual dimensions are connected, various socio-economic and cultural factors affect individual wellness quite differently. In most instances, alcohol use is linked to transgenerational trauma and the residential school system; this has had negative impacts on Indigenous peoples' states of well-being resulting in negative social capital (Portes, 1998). Negative social capital was first introduced by Portes and Landolt (1996) in "The Downside of Social Capital," which provides a rationale as to why social capital is linked to healthy and vibrant communities but also holds downsides (Portes & Landolt, 1996). In a later work, Portes and Landolt (2000) conclude that "social capital of any significance can seldom be acquired without the investment of some material resources and the possession of some cultural knowledge, enabling the individual to establish relations with valued others" (p. 533). What this implies is that social capital, in terms of bridging and bonding, can be a "powerful force promoting group projects but, as noted previously, it consists of the ability to marshal resources through social networks, not the resources themselves" (Portes & Landolt, 2000, p. 546). Given that social capital is a hypothesis that involves multilevel analysis (individual, family, community, and nation), it has been a useful empirical analysis in understanding the ways in which individual and community well-being are linked by way of employment, income levels, education attainments, and also traditional and cultural activities. Bourdieu (1993) sees the family as the main site of accumulation and transmission of social capital, which fits well when we consider the cultural transmission of negative forms of social capital. The results of the study have empirically shown how alcohol use, residential school attendance, transgenerational trauma, food insecurity, and inadequate housing also impact dimensions of Indigenous health and wellness.

One of the main questions I posed at the onset of this book is "How is the FNPOW related to a decolonizing process and does the FNPOW generate determinants of health and wellness that advance self-determination?" This is an important question and remains inadequately addressed in the literature. To answer this question, I focused on decolonizing of research methods to trace the historical development of the FNPOW to garner an understanding of how and why it was created; I also explored the myriad of ways it is used by FNHA. In doing so, I learned about the impacts of transgenerational trauma, family networks, alcohol consumption, and Indigenous traditional and cultural activities as well as other social and economic factors on individual and community levels of well-being. By applying a decolonizing research framework and a strengths-based Indigenous perspective using the FNPOW, the results of this study demonstrate that participation in Indigenous cultural activities is in and of itself an everyday act of resurgence that serves to support Indigenous peoples to move towards building resilience and resources that have positive impacts on spiritual, physical, emotional, and mental wellness (Corntassel, 2012). According to Kovach (2009), decolonization is a "bridge between two worlds" and is a place where non-Indigenous researchers and anti-oppressive strategies can be allies for Indigenous methodologies by "making space for Indigenous methods ... protocols, ethics, data collection processes" (p. 86).

Critical Reflections

Allyship and Solidarity

Structures of inequality result in oppression, and when we think about it, we all have been complicit in the oppression of another person at some point (Bishop, 2015). We are encompassed by oppressive mentalities, which for Bishop are similar to the air we breathe (Bishop, 2015).

Becoming an ally is necessary for breaking the cycle of oppression and starts with understanding your own privilege and positionality in society (Bishop, 2015). Oppression is linked to allyship, which we can apply to processes such as decolonization and to community-engaged research practices when we consider the ways in which we benefit from settler colonialism. In her book *On Becoming an Ally: Breaking the Cycle of Oppression in People* (2002), Anne Bishop explains that all settlers do not benefit equally from the settler-colonial state, nor did many people settle of their own free will. There are systems of oppression such as slavery, hetero-patriarchy, white supremacy, and market imperialism that are embedded in a neoliberal capitalist class economy that are the direct result of colonization. For Bishop, six steps are involved in becoming an ally: (1) understanding oppression, how it came about, how it is held in place, and how it stamps its pattern on individuals and institutions that continually recreate it; (2) understanding different oppressions, how they are similar, how they differ, and how they reinforce one another; (3) understanding consciousness and healing; (4) becoming a worker for your own liberation; (5) becoming an ally; and (6) maintaining hope (Bishop, 2002). Bishop argues that being an ally involves understanding oppressive structural processes, addressing what she refers to as "liberal individualism" embedded in neoliberal capitalist social organization (Bishop, 2002). The process of becoming an ally must not be out of guilt but must be an active role in supporting the contesting of the colonization process by Indigenous peoples.

Other authors have expressed the importance of how allies should act and behave in terms of anti-oppressive strategies in challenging macro social structures of power and white supremacy. The article "Accomplices Not Allies: Abolishing the Ally Industrial Complex" examines how the commodification and exploitation of allyship is a growing trend in the activism community. It is crucial to identify points of intervention against the ally industrial complex and focus on becoming an accomplice to Indigenous peoples as opposed to looking for ways that allies use their position of power for personal gain and benefit. Algonquin Anishinaabe-kwe scholar Lynn Gehl's *Ally Bill of Responsibilities* (n.d.) outlines sixteen responsibilities for settlers where she characterizes ally performance based in having a knowledge of one's own ancestral history and awareness of one's own privilege. For Gehl it is crucial to listen and reflect while accepting the responsibility of being an ally and while ensuring that you do not usurp space and resources in the act of being a responsible ally. Thus, being an ally in the context of a research process means making a sincere effort to transform the researcher–participant relationship beyond a colonial mentality that reifies the power structures of knowledge generation to that of sharing "power-with" the people who may be affected by the findings (Wallace, 2011). However, such an approach can be mistaken for a recipe of what makes an effective ally.

For Walia (2012), being an ally is conflated with power and it is problematic when used as a form of self-identification, a badge of honour, or an accomplishment. Walia (2012) argues that corporate wealth is largely based on subsidies gained from theft of Indigenous lands and resources and the devastating assimilation of Indigenous peoples' cultures and traditions. As settlers, we must consider ourselves beneficiaries of the illegal settlement of Indigenous people's lands; therefore, building long-term relationships of solidarity can only happen through a sustained ongoing commitment (Walia, 2012). The work on being an ally and creating solidarity helps us to understand that there are important differences "in being" an ally when compared to "the doing" of allyship. Allyship is a process of continual learning, listening, and personal growth (Bishop, 2002; Gehl, n.d.; Walia, 2012). I argue that allyship is a relational process in that it is practised by the researcher in relation to community and involves an ongoing, continuous attempt to create meaningful relationships; otherwise, it runs the risk of reifying the power structures of oppression that the work intends to challenge and change. This can happen because people can abuse their power and privilege by creating titles, hierarchies, and labels of identification that serve to perpetuate power imbalances. To work in allyship is different than simply recognizing ones' own privilege situated in society's structures of injustice. Allyship is not about assuming a label and then carrying out associated role performance and expected behaviours that are associated with that label. Part of becoming an ally is also recognizing one's own experience of oppression; becoming an ally in research means understanding that allyship is a process. Through this process we seek to understand, honour, and centre Indigenous ethical protocols in all aspects of the research design process.

Relational Allyship and Responsive Research

I have been working in community for almost two decades to generate knowledge that is based in culturally responsive and relevant practices. In my teachings of research methodologies and more recently from a decolonizing standpoint, I have been asked an important question: "If decolonization is related to self-determination and Indigenous scholars advocate for Indigenous resurgence then how do I, as a settler-ally, participate in these processes of Indigenous resurgence?" Anishinaabe scholar Leanne Simpson's recent book *As We Have Always Done* is clear in advocating that cultural resurgence is a practice rooted in Indigenous thinking but also political activism. Understanding it from this lens creates a place for inclusion, a place where all of us together reject the settler colonial state, along with heteropatriarchy, white supremacy, and neoliberal capitalist systems of oppression (Simpson, 2017). For me, I would like to answer this question by sharing my own experiences in participating in Indigenous ceremonies and activities by invitation. I consider it an honour to be part of these ceremonies and I am grateful for this gifting. I don't base my research methods in ceremony but what I do offer is a process of holding space to bear witness to these Indigenous resurgence practices. I am relationally accountable to the peoples and communities I work with and for.

In this book I have described how a mixed methods participatory study can illustrate how the ongoing structures of colonialization continue to negatively impact health and wellness of Indigenous peoples in urban centres across Canada. The decolonizing strategies that I used were (1) critiquing Western knowledge production and the measures of health and wellness and its effects; (2) using the FNPOW-centred Indigenous knowledge systems to produce determinants of health and wellness that are anchored in Indigenous world views as a form of resurgence of Indigenous knowledge that will benefit the community; (3) honouring Indigenous ethical protocols through a research agreement with the FNHA; and (4) embodying self-identification and allyship. These decolonizing research strategies support two key mandates of the FNHA. which are to "incorporate and promote First Nations knowledge, beliefs, values, practices, medicines and models of health and healing into the First Nations Health Programs, recognizing that these may be reflected differently in different regions of BC" (FNHA, 2016c, p. 1) and to ensure the results of the study have "carried out research and policy development in the area of First Nations health and wellness" (FNHA, 2016, p. 1).

Recall that the objective of a decolonizing approach is not to "discard all theory or Western knowledge" (Smith, 1999, p. 39); rather, decolonizing methodologies draw from existing knowledge and bridge western and Indigenous knowledge systems through a two-eyed seeing approach. Decolonizing research advocates a *re*-searching, re-righting, and remembering of knowledge using a strengths-based approach to do research that builds on Indigenous knowledge and requires a change in conceptualizations of the research process and requires the development of new paradigms and different ways of thinking about and doing research (Corntassel, 2012; Kovach, 2005, 2009; Simpson, 2011; Smith, 1999, 2006, 2012). Resistance is about challenging colonial impositions while resurgence is about regenerating knowledge and land-based practices. Resistance and resurgence are necessary components to foster Mino-Bimaadiziwin because they honour and support Indigenous world views with a holistic approach to the good life with an emphasis on culture and tradition.

In future research, if we are to accurately describe the determinants of Indigenous health and wellness, the research must be contextualized in transgenerational trauma and also wellness practices such as land-based traditions and cultural activities. In addition, these determinants need to be linked to specific historical, cultural, political, social, and economic contexts that must be accurately documented. Research designs need to be culturally responsive, which means that researchers need to work in partnership with Indigenous peoples, communities, and/or organizations in a way that avoids misinterpretations and misrepresentations in the knowledge inquiry process. This will support the generation of research findings that are anchored in Indigenous knowledge systems and accurate cross-cultural representations, producing estimates of population health that are better equipped to inform recommendations for health, healing, and well-being. These are the types of new relationships that will facilitate reconciliation because Indigenous peoples, communities, and organizations can re-story the historical trauma on a number of levels and create new ways of understanding and contesting the deeply ingrained structures of inequality.

Another important research question posed at the onset of this study asked, "How does understanding well-being through a decolonizing research approach support an understanding of well-being that can be of direct benefit to urban Indigenous peoples?" This is also directly related to social capital when we consider that we are living in an era of reconciliation. All new relationships between Indigenous peoples and the Canadian government, and non-Indigenous peoples for that matter, will continue to act as a social determinant of health and wellness until we acknowledge and develop empirically based indicators of social relationships to include within Indigenous health analysis. This will require an investigation of contemporary relationships and an understanding of Indigenous sovereignty issues, whereby the FNHA as a self-determined health organization is exemplary. Incorporating this knowledge with theories on social capital in health analysis needs to be further developed to provide a method to identify indicators of relationships that contribute to the health and wellness of Indigenous peoples. This study is a first step in that direction and has shown how we can build bridges between knowledge systems of different ontological origins using multi-epistemological methods of sociological inquiry. That being said, I have also come to realize that two-eyed seeing has several limitations that I think responsive research is better able to address.

Responsive Research, the TRAC Method, and Indigenous Data Sovereignty

What does it mean to decolonize research? In "Unsettling Settler Colonialism: The Discourse and Politics of Settlers, and Solidarity with Indigenous Nations," Snelgrove et al. make the point that centring Indigenous peoples' articulations is critical to deploying a relational approach to settler colonial power and that practices of solidarity will otherwise reify settler colonialisms and other modes of domination (Snelgrove et al., 2014, pp. 7–9). To decolonize research is an everyday practice that involves the critique of conventional epistemologies and dominant knowledge systems to create culturally respectful frameworks that do not place the value of western ways of understanding over Indigenous ways of knowing. According to Kwakwaka'wakw scholar Sarah Hunt and Cindy Holmes (2015), "While large-scale actions such as rallies, protests and blockades are frequently acknowledged as sites of resistance, the daily actions undertaken by individual Indigenous people, families, and communities often go unacknowledged but are no less vital to decolonial processes" (pp. 157–8). By looking at the everyday, we gain a deeper sense of how relationality, responsibility, and personal decolonization are embodied and practised within a research context. For Indigenous peoples, ongoing colonial policies and practices aimed at eroding cultural identity and the legacy of the residential school system have led other scholars to conclude that severe historical trauma has, as a consequence, been passed through the generations (Brave Heart, 2014; Brave Heart & DeBruyn, 1998; Gone et al., 2014; Maté, 2008; Ross, 1996) and that the legacy of the residential schools still has an impact on individuals, families, and communities today. There are varied uses of the terms to describe trauma in the Indigenous literature, and in some instances the term *intergenerational trauma* is used to explain the transmission of trauma from one generation to the next while *historical trauma* has also been ubiquitous (Brave Heart, 2014; Gagné, 1998; Gone et al., 2014). Indigenous scholars and trauma experts Brave Heart and Debruyn (1998) argue that "Like children of Jewish Holocaust survivors, subsequent generations of American Indians also have a pervasive sense of pain from what happened to their ancestors" (p. 64). Similarly, Gone et al. (2014) have invited us to rethink the term *historical trauma* by making linkages using historical trauma research with survivors of the Holocaust to identify a comparable cluster of events correlated with massive group trauma across generations. "In seeking to understand the transgenerational effects of historical trauma and processes of recovery, some Indigenous scholars and mental health practitioners have made explicit analogies to the Holocaust and its health impacts on the Jewish people" (Gone et al., 2014, p. 301). The study findings presented in this book have shown that Indigenous peoples experience individual trauma and communities experience collective trauma. The specific terminology of trauma directly pertains to understanding the impacts of trauma when working with Indigenous peoples (Gone et al., 2014).

Understanding how trauma and extractive research processes enhance trauma is an ethical requirement of doing research work with Indigenous peoples. For example, in this book transgenerational trauma is discussed extensively in the findings and framed the research scope, design, and ethical manner by which this work was carried out. With multiple generations of Indigenous peoples and communities having been affected by residential schools, the ongoing trauma affects the economic, social, and political structures in communities and has consequences for systems of dependency and marginalization. At the individual level, we would expect consequences that include increased anxiety, increased stress, and increased use of alcohol (Gagné, 1998; Helin, 2006).

Given the complexity of transgenerational trauma for Indigenous peoples, it is clear that "disrupting the intergenerational transmission of trauma will require holistic and multifaceted approaches to improving health and well-being ... there is a deep shame that is felt by many Aboriginal people that is linked to the processes of colonialism" (Aguiar & Halseth, 2015, p. 23). This shame is felt by individuals, families, communities, and Nations. In order to re-establish a sense of pride in Indigenous identity for individuals and communities and to effectively deal with unresolved trauma, there is now an emphasis on "culture as treatment" activities (Gone, 2013 as cited in Aguiar & Halseth, 2015, p. 23). Research into resilience and Indigenous resurgence has shown that the sense of historical rootedness Indigenous peoples have and maintain through cultural activities helps them cope with issues created through colonization (Alfred & Corntassel, 2005; Gone, 2011; Gone & Kirmayer, 2010: Kelley et al., 2012; Kirmayer et al., 2011, 2012; Kral, 2012; Reading et al., 2007). Ties to land, culture, and community are essential for survivance, which is "an active sense of presence over absence, deracination, and oblivion" (Vizenor, 2007, p. 3).

Two-eyed seeing offers a way to decolonize research methods and has been widely used in the field of health research. The principle of two-eyed seeing utilizes the strengths of western scientific knowledge and the strengths of Indigenous knowledges to weave back and forth between world views to find the most applicable fit for research (Bartlett et al., 2012). This weaving process gives way to its integrative approach to understanding health and wellness research but is not without limitations. First, it does not actually integrate western methods with Indigenous methods at each stage of the research design process and project life cycle. In turn, this guiding principle of differing world views that run parallel to each other is not as integrative as a braiding method. It is this concept of using two world views, which has also been described by other authors as a way of bringing together of Indigenous and mainstream knowledges (see Archibald, 2008; Kovach, 2009; Wilson, 2008), that enables a researcher to move between world views. Two-eyed seeing was a useful analytical approach for the study I presented in this book because I was able to weave a case study framework with oral histories based in Indigenous storytelling as a way of seeing health outcomes differently.

The Limitations of Two-eyed Seeing

The limitations of two-eyed seeing became apparent to me during community-driven research processes on several different projects. One of the limitations I have noted is that two-eyed seeing is more of a principle than a method per se. It is not trauma-informed, which renders it problematic when working in community and given the nature of research topics such as understanding impacts of resources, development projects, and gendered violence. Two-eyed seeing does not braid Indigenous and western epistemologies together at specific stages in the research process (e.g., research scoping, data collection, data processing, interpretation, and writing), which poses difficulties with praxis. With decades of community-driven research experience between the two of us, Cherokee scholar Jeff Corntassel and I advocate for responsive research and we see it as offering more than a scientific notion of "research responsive to public needs" (Bud, 2014). Responsive research and the Translocal Relationships, Relational Accountability Accountability Mechanisms Community Timeframes (TRAC) method emerged while we worked on different community-based projects nationally and internationally and we see it as an approach that braids Indigenous and western social scientific epistemologies at each stage of the research process. Responsive research facilitates meaningful forms of relational accountability in community partnerships where research programs are responsive to the short- and long-term goals of Indigenous Nations and peoples. Responsive research emerged in community-based projects when we realized that the main qualitative tools were insufficient (Quinless & Corntassel, 2018). We support Indigenous peoples in the process of owning their community information. We believe that research processes for Indigenous peoples by Indigenous peoples is an important step in self-determination and governance (Quinless & Corntassel, 2018). During our work we applied responsive research in accordance with the following principles:

1. Indigenous communities should work in partnership with researchers to generate their own community knowledge.
2. Throughout the process Indigenous communities should have control of research and data collection processes through agreed-on informed, free, and prior consent.

So how does responsive research fit with other qualitative research traditions? There are five main qualitative traditions used in social science research: phenomenology, ethnography, narrative research, case study, and grounded theory. All can fall under the umbrella of participatory action methods. Participatory action research differs from most other approaches to Indigenous health and wellness research because it is based in the co-creation of knowledge and action with the intention of reducing health inequities through community partnerships and people who are committed to improving their own health and well-being (Absolon & Willett, 2005; Ahenakew, 2012; Castellano, 2004; Corntasell 2008, 2012; Kovach 2005, 2009; Quinless, 2017; Smith, 1999; Wilson, 2008). While aspects of these methods are useful, they have not been approached from a trauma-informed and decolonized lens and have the following five significant limitations that have proven ineffective for some community-driven research projects:

(1) PAR methods are not sufficiently culturally informed and community driven.
(2) PAR methods are not guided by community ethical protocols.
(3) PAR methods do not use a trauma-informed lens.
(4) PAR methods do not provide a strengths-based approach to data generation.
(5) Data curation and digital sovereignty are not adequately introduced into the research design phases of the project.

Through various research projects, we have centred Indigenous ways of knowing through all phases of the research design process. By decolonizing our research activities, we have *re*-searched knowledge using a strengths-based and trauma-informed approach to these practices. Understanding community ethical protocols has been an important part of how we have been building on Indigenous knowledge (Quinless & Corntassel, 2018). This required a change in conceptualizations of the research process and the development of new paradigms (Corntassel, 2012; Kovach, 2005, 2009; Simpson, 2011; Smith 1999, 2006, 2012) and different ways of thinking about and doing research.

We identify five main tenets of an approach to responsive research through the TRAC method that are guided by community ethical protocols and can be applied when working within an Indigenous context.

(1) The TRAC method has emerged through successful community partnerships with an understanding and response to applying a trauma-informed research practice.

(2) It centres community knowledge and focuses on sustainability of knowledge.

(3) It braids western sociological methods with Indigenous methodologies.

(4) It approaches research from strengths and is not a deficit model.

(5) It incorporates interpretative flexibility, which means using standard research tools with components that reflect cultural diversity and meanings and interpretations anchored in Indigenous ways of knowing, seeing, and understanding (Quinless & Corntassel, 2018).

The TRAC method of responsive research is based in four approaches (identified below) that braid together western methodologies with Indigenous methodologies into different stages of the research design life cycle.

(1) **Translocal relationships** are relationships developed that respect diversity by focusing on localized Indigenous knowledge and place with the intention of developing sustainable, long-term relationships that are mutually beneficial. Future Indigenous Nation relationships emanate from your localized partnerships. This is a useful design when working with various communities in vast geographic regions because it accounts for the specific community contexts at the micro level that can radiate out to other communities.

(2) **Relational accountability** is our ethical responsibility to research. Research partnerships and collaborations are generated in conversation with and by ongoing goals of Indigenous Nations. Finding culturally relevant ways of implementing free, prior, and informed consent is especially important here.

(3) **Accountability mechanisms** honour Indigenous Nations
protocols and practices throughout the research design process
and research partnership. This is what we do with the information
we have been given and a reminder that the research processes
that we engage in are just as important as the outcome of the
project. Having continuous communication and processes for
renewing our commitment of the project will keep the project on
track. These outcomes can be integrated into the data processing
and interpretation phases of the project and also into writing of
the report and knowledge sharing back to the community in ways
that will be useful to the community.

(4) **Community timeframes** is a way of honouring the fact that
Indigenous Nations have their own sense of time based on place-
based relationships, language, ceremonies, familial responsibilities,
kinship networks, and sacred living histories (Corntassel, 2008,
2012). As a researcher, it is important that you adhere to the
community's sense of time versus imposing your own deadlines
and needs. The challenges to completing key informant interviews
include the fact that they can take a significant amount of time
to complete (i.e., scheduling and rescheduling) and findings
from interviews can be challenging to analyse and synthesize
(i.e., different stakeholder groups with differing levels of program
involvement, differing agendas, and differing understandings of
and experiences with the program).

Figure 6 is a display of the TRAC approach that emerged during
several community-driven research projects at different stages in the
research process. Each of the four quadrants outlines widely accepted
practices of research stages that are common among qualitative
researchers using social scientific methods and from textbooks that
I use to teach qualitative research methods in the discipline of sociology (Ritchie et al., 2013). These stages are Stage 1: Research Objectives
and Framing; Stage 2: Research Design; Stage 3: Data Collection; and
Stage 4: Knowledge Sharing with the necessary research tasks associated with each stage in the research life cycle.

The TRAC method was developed in response to inadequacies in
integrating social scientific and Indigenous methodologies simultaneously. It is reflective of a decolonized standpoint to narrowly defined
social science methods and provides more of an integrative research
approach compared to two-eyed seeing. While working in various
communities, Dr. Corntassel and I realized that, in order to braid
Indigenous and western knowledge systems, the following needed to

Figure 6. Responsive research and the TRAC method

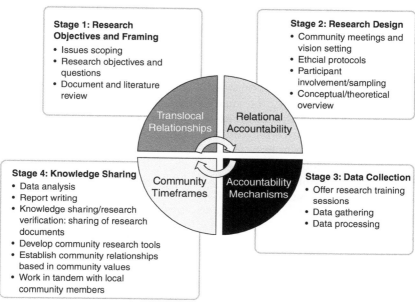

Stage 1: Research Objectives and Framing
- Issues scoping
- Research objectives and questions
- Document and literature review

Stage 2: Research Design
- Community meetings and vision setting
- Ethcial protocols
- Participant involvement/sampling
- Conceptual/theoretical overview

Stage 4: Knowledge Sharing
- Data analysis
- Report writing
- Knowledge sharing/research verification: sharing of research documents
- Develop community research tools
- Establish community relationships based in community values
- Work in tandem with local community members

Stage 3: Data Collection
- Offer research training sessions
- Data gathering
- Data processing

Translocal Relationships

Relational Accountability

Community Timeframes

Accountability Mechanisms

Source: Quinless & Corntassel, 2018.

occur at various stages of the research process and we carried out the following:

- Using a trauma-informed approach in which we held space to witness and listen to participants through compassionate and empathic techniques while gathering data in each of the communities
- Modifying standardized research language (metadata standards) to better relate to Indigenous world views. For example, we changed *data collection* to *data gathering* and *database* to *data tracker*, along with many other research terminologies that were better aligned with Indigenous world views
- Developing meaningful partnerships by supporting community initiatives through out-of-pocket expenses. For example, we have supported local artists; gifted passes for children to attend recreational activities where funds were not available; provided soccer equipment to children living in the communities of Jinijini and Akropong in Ghana as requested to support community

wellness; and ensured traditional foods be provided at research
events, which was incredibly important in respecting community
protocols around notions of sharing and healing
- Infusing the research process with culturally informed and
  ethically guided practice by centring Indigenous-specific
  knowledge, which requires us to decolonize various stages of the
  research process. We responsively work on Indigenous timelines
  and reschedule interviews when needed, we engage in several
  informal conversations to build relationship, and we participate in
  ceremonial activities when invited
- Looking to the community to identify its strengths in regard to
  health and well-being and healing from violence
- Supporting development of capacity by providing research
  knowledge training to build knowledge capacity among
  community research staff. We have created customized research
  tools (data tracking systems) and gifted them to community-based
  organizations and Band offices and administration to support
  future work endeavours such as grant and proposal writing and
  business development

Again, the TRAC method of responsive research emerged from a
community-driven research project and is based in four approaches that
braid western methodologies with Indigenous methods and include
(1) translocal relationships, (2) relational accountability, (3) accountability mechanisms, and (4) community timeframes. There is currently
considerable interest inside but also outside of the academy in a range
of issues associated with decolonizing research methods and Indigenizing health and wellness. It is our wish that this initial discussion of
responsive research using the TRAC method will be beneficial in this
regard.

Indigenous Data Sovereignty

In May 2016, Canada officially signed UNDRIP and began an attempt
to harmonize Canadian law with the standards set in the declaration.[1]
This along with the ninety-four Calls to Action of the 2015 Truth and
Reconciliation (TRC) are two strong instruments of reconciliation that
centre free, prior, and informed consent, which has direct impacts
on data gathering. But the methods and arrangements for gathering,

---

1 For example, see https://openparliament.ca/bills/42-1/C-262/

processing, and sharing data are not clear. The approach of many government departments and academic institutions is to work with Indigenous communities and organizations to coordinate Indigenous and tripartite initiatives and strategies to forge new relationships. In moving forward with reconciliation it is critical that we unsettle conversations to think more reflectively on how the data rights and interests of Indigenous peoples are secured. Responsive research through the TRAC methodology supports Indigenous data sovereignty (IDS), which seeks to protect Indigenous knowledge that is based on Indigenous peoples', communities', and Nations' own terms. In Canada, IDS movements have already been established through the FNIGC research data practices based in the principles outlined through OCAP, which is trademarked through FNIGC and supported by the FNHA. The FNIGC has provided momentum to the IDS movement in recognizing the rights of Indigenous peoples to govern the collection, ownership, and dissemination of their own knowledge (data). This is based in an Indigenous rights framework in accordance with international declarations such as UNDRIP and acknowledgment of Indigenous peoples' inherent right to govern their people, lands, and knowledge.

The ideas presented in this book centre decolonizing research methods into mainstream sociology in a way that has until now been neglected. I have explained how research design practices need to be culturally responsive, which means that researchers need to work in partnership with Indigenous peoples, communities, and/or organizations so as to avoid misinterpretations and misrepresentations in the knowledge inquiry process. This will support the generation of research findings that are anchored in Indigenous knowledge systems, world views, epistemologies, ontologies, and axiology.

I have explained how various mechanisms of the current colonial system explicitly define and frame questions of well-being – how well-being should be conceptualized, measured, and evaluated for Indigenous peoples – thus failing to integrate Indigenous knowledge systems and world views about health and wellness. This colonial knowledge system has been internalized by many Indigenous communities and peoples, which further colonizes their inner life-worlds (Browne et al., 2005) and serves to validate thinking about and to support a colonial mentality (Alfred, 2008) about what does and what does not constitute Indigenous wellness. The findings in this book come from applying what Alberta Marshall, Elder of the Eskasoni First Nation, refers to as a two-eyed way of seeing health and wellness within an urban context. Two-eyed seeing is uses Indigenous knowledge systems and western-based knowledge systems to provide a holistic lens to understanding health and wellness (Iwama et al., 2009). It draws on social capital analysis, western social thinking, and notions of becoming an ally (Bishop, 2015) when thinking about wellness with Indigenous ways of understanding being-well through the FNPOW. While previous scholars have written extensively about the devastating impacts of colonizing research processes on Indigenous peoples and communities (Ahenakew, 2011; Baskin, 2005; Chandler & Lalonde, 1998; Cooke et al., 2008; Drabsch, 2012; Hill & Cooke, 2014; Gone, 2011; Gone & Kirmayer, 2010; Kelley et al., 2012; Kirmayer et al., 2011, 2012; Kovach, 2005, 2009; Kral, 2012; Lawson-Te Aho & Liu, 2010; Loppie-Reading & Wien, 2009; Mundel & Chapman, 2010; Quinless, 2015; Smith, 1999; White, Beavon, et al., 2007; White, Wingert, et al., 2007; White et al., 2009; Wilson & Rosenberg, 2002), I am seeking ways to engage in unsettling conversations in order to provide further insights about the everyday ways that we engage in discourse around Indigenous health and well-being.

Decolonizing research is an ongoing journey through a series of the unseen ways of acting on relationships through language, stories, and ceremony that regenerate Indigenous ways of life. Decolonization is the process of regaining self-determination and social, economic, cultural, and political independence (Corntassel, 2012). Tuck and Yang (2012) also explain that decolonization is not a metaphor but brings about meaningful relationships that focus on the repatriation of Indigenous lands and life. Smith (2012) further emphasizes that addressing power structures and dynamics in research is important in understanding self-determination and a critical step in decolonizing methodologies. This is because it is often white settlers who imposed their own views, narratives, and assumptions upon Indigenous experiences and culture (Smith, 2012). The decolonization of research methods in the context of individual and community health and wellness is a growing, interdisciplinary field.

While I wrote this book predominantly from a sociological perspective and using a two-eyed seeing approach, the approach has also incorporated historical research and a cultural studies approach and has discussed topics related to social work, gender studies, and political science. This book would be useful to scholars, practitioners, and graduate students across a range of social science and humanities disciplines but the book can also have widespread appeal to those outside of academia who are interested in applied research. As researchers, we can strive for better ways to work in relational allyship, to bear witness to these research processes, and to support innovative ways of understanding that contest the deeply ingrained structures of inequality that have galvanized western thinking and research practices. I believe this book is an initial step in unsettling conversations about research praxis and a positive step along a pathway forward that requires ongoing commitments to processes of decolonizing research methodologies. Unsettling conversations about *what we know* and *how we do* social research open space for forging new relationships that will facilitate positive research relationships between researchers and Indigenous peoples, communities, and organizations.

References

Abele, F. (2004). *Urgent need, serious opportunity: Towards a new social model for Canada's Aboriginal peoples.* Ottawa: Canadian Policy Research Networks. Canadian Electronic Library/desLibris.

Aboriginal Affairs Working Group. (2010). *A framework for action in education, economic development and violence against Aboriginal women and girls.* Aboriginal Affairs Working Report to Premiers. Available at https://www2.gov.bc.ca/assets/gov/environment/natural-resource-stewardship/consulting-with-first-nations/first-nations/report_aboriginal_affairs_working_group.pdf

Absolon, K.E. (2011). *Kaandossiwin: How we come to know.* Fernwood Publishing.

Absolon, K.E., & Willett, C. (2005). Putting ourselves forward: Location in Aboriginal research. In L.A. Brown (Ed.), *Research as resistance: Critical, Indigenous and anti-oppressive approaches* (pp. 97–126). Canadian Scholars' Press.

Aguiar, W., & Halseth, R. (2015). *Aboriginal peoples and historic trauma: The processes of intergenerational transmission.* National Collaborating Centre for Aboriginal Health (NCCAH). Available at http://www.ccnsa-nccah.ca/docs/context/RPT-HistoricTrauma-IntergenTransmission-Aguiar-Halseth-EN.pdf

Ahenakew, C. (2011). The birth of the "Windigo": The construction of Aboriginal health in biomedical and traditional Indigenous models of medicine. *Critical Literacies: Theories and Practices, 5*(1), 3–13.

Ahenakew, C. (2012). *The effects of historical trauma, community capacity and place of residence on the self-reported health of Canada's Indigenous population* [Unpublished doctoral dissertation]. University of Calgary.

Alfred, G.R. (1995). *Heeding the voices of our ancestors.* Oxford University Press.

Alfred, T. (2005). *Wasase: Indigenous pathways of action and freedom.* Broadview Press.

Alfred, T. (2008). *Peace, power, righteousness: An Indigenous manifesto*. Oxford University Press.

Alfred, T. (2009). Colonialism and state dependency. *Journal de la santé autochtone, 5*(3), 42–60.

Alfred, T., & Corntassel, J. (2005). Being Indigenous: Resurgences against contemporary colonialism. *Government and Opposition, 40*(4), 597–614.

Aman, C. (2008). Aboriginal students and school mobility in British Columbia public schools. *Alberta Journal of Educational Research, 54*(4), 365–77.

Anaquot, K. (2006). *Measuring progress: Program evaluation. Final report of the Aboriginal Healing Foundation* (Vol. II). Aboriginal Healing Foundation.

Andersen, C. (2014). *Métis: Race, recognition, and the struggle for Indigenous peoplehood*. UBC Press.

Andersen, C., & Walter, M. (2014). *Indigenous statistics: A quantitative research guide*. Left Coast Press.

Anderson, K. (2001). *A recognition of being: Reconstructing native womanhood* (2nd ed.). Women's Press.

Andreotti, V., Ahenakew, C., & Cooper, G. (2011). Epistemological pluralism: Ethical and pedagogical challenges in higher education. *Alter-Natives: An International Journal of Indigenous Peoples, 7*(1), 40–50.

Antonovsky, A. (1996). The salutogenic model as a theory to guide health promotion. *Health Promotion International, 11*(1), 11–18.

Apparurai, A. (1993). Numbers in the colonial imagination. In C.A. Breckebridge and P. van der Veer (Eds.), *Orientalism and the postcolonial predicament* (pp. 314–49). University of Pennsylvania Press.

Archibald, J. (2008). *Indigenous storywork: Educating the heart, mind, body, and spirit*. UBC Press.

Archibald, L. (2006). *Promising healing practices in Aboriginal communities. Final report of the Aboriginal Healing Foundation* (Vol. III). Aboriginal Healing Foundation.

Armstrong, R.P. (2001). *The geographical patterns of socio-economic well-being of First Nations communities in Canada*. Agriculture and Rural Working Paper Series, Working Paper No. 46. Statistics Canada.

Ashcroft, B., Griffiths, G., & Tiffin, H. (2007). *Postcolonial studies: The key concepts*. Routledge.

Australian Bureau of Statistics. (2016). *Measures of Australia's progress, 2010*. Retrieved from http://www.abs.gov.au/ausstats/abs@.nsf/Lookup/by%20Subject/1370.0~2010~Chapter~Future%20directions%20%20(7)

Bang, M., Curley, L., Kessel, A., Marin, A, Suzukovich, E.S., III, & Strack, G. (2014). Muskrat theories, tobacco in the streets, and living Chicago as Indigenous land. *Environmental Education Research, 20*(1), 37–55. https://doi.org/10.1080/13504622.2013.865113

Bartlett, C., Marshall, M., & Marshall, A. (2012). Two-eyed seeing and other lessons learned within a co-learning journey of bringing together Indigenous and mainstream knowledges and ways of knowing. *Journal of Environmental Studies and Sciences, 2*(4), 331–40. https://doi.org/10.1007/s13412-012-0086-8

Baskin, C. (2005). *Circles of inclusion: Aboriginal world views in social work education* (458721743) [Doctoral dissertation, University of Toronto]. Library and Archives Canada.

Bastien, B. (2004). *Blackfoot ways of knowing. The worldview of the Siksikaitsitapi.* University of Calgary Press.

Bastien, B., Kremer, J., Kuokkanen, R., & Vickers, P. (2003). Healing the impact of colonization, genocide, and racism on Indigenous populations. In S. Kripper & T. McIntyre (Eds.), *The psychological impact of war trauma on civilians: An international perspective* (pp. 25–37). Praeger Publishers.

Baum, C. (2007). *The effects of food stamps on obesity.* Contractor and Cooperator Report No. 34. U.S. Department of Agriculture, Economic Research Service.

Baum, F. (1998). Communities, participation and social capital. In F. Baum (Ed.), *The new public health: An Australian perspective* (pp. 93–9). Oxford University Press.

BC Progress Board. (2010). 10th Annual Benchmark Report. Retrieved from https://www.cbc.ca/bc/news/bc-101216-progress-board-report.pdf

Beatty, B., & Weber-Beeds, A. (2011). Mitho-Pimatisiwin for the elderly: The strength of a shared caregiving approach in Aboriginal health. In D. Newhouse, K. FitzMaurice, T. McGuire-Adams, & D. Jetté (Eds.), *Well-being in the Aboriginal community: Fostering Biimaadiziwin, a national research conference on urban Aboriginal Peoples* (pp. 113–30). Thompson Educational Publishing.

Beavon, D., & Jetté, D. (2009). Journeys of a generation: Broadening the Indigenous wellbeing policy research agenda. *Canadian Issues,* Winter.

Berkman, L.F., & Kawachi, I. (2000). *Social epidemiology.* Oxford University Press.

Billings, J., & Hashem, F. (2009, April 10*). Salutogenesis and the promotion of positive mental health in older people* [Literature review]. Mental Health and Well-being in Older People – Making it Happen, Madrid. https://www.mscbs.gob.es/organizacion/sns/planCalidadSNS/docs/saludmental/conference_report__en.pdf

Bishop, A. (2002). *Becoming an ally: Breaking the cycle of oppression* (2nd ed.). Fernwood Publishing.

Bishop, A. (2015). *Becoming an ally: Breaking the cycle of oppression* (3rd ed.). Fernwood Publishing.

Bishop, R. (2005). Freeing ourselves from neocolonial domination in research: A Kaupapa Māori approach to creating knowledge. In N.K. Denzin & Y.S. Lincoln (Eds.), *Handbook of qualitative research* (3rd ed., pp. 109–38). Sage Publications.

Blackstock, C. (2007). Residential schools: Did they really close or just morph into child welfare? *Indigenous Law Journal, 6*(1), 71–8.

Blackstock, C. (2009). The occasional evil of angels: Learning from the experiences of Aboriginal peoples and social work. *First Peoples Child and Family Review, 4*(1), 28–37.

Blackstock, C. (2012). Reconciliation means not saying sorry twice: Lessons from child welfare in Canada. In Rogers, S., DeGagné, M., Dewar, J., & Lowry, G. (Eds.), *Speaking my truth: Reflections on reconciliation and residential schools* (pp. 163–75). Aboriginal Healing Foundation.

Blackstock, C., Trocme, N., & Bennett, M. (2004). Child maltreatment investigations among Aboriginal and non-Aboriginal families in Canada. *Violence against Women, 10*(5), 1–16.

Blishen, B., Carroll, W., & Moore, C. (1987). The 1981 socioeconomic index for occupations in Canada. *Review of Sociology and Anthropology, 4*.

Bourdieu, P. (1972). *Outline of a theory of practice.* Cambridge University Press.

Bourdieu, P. (1984). *Distinction: A social critique of the judgement of taste.* (Richard Nice, Trans.) Harvard University Press. (Original work published 1979).

Bourdieu, P. (1986). The forms of capital. In J. Richardson (Ed.), *Handbook of theory and research for the sociology of education* (pp. 241–58). Greenwood Press.

Bourdieu, P. (1993). *The field of cultural production: Essays on art and literature.* Polity Books.

Bourdieu, P., & Wacquant, L. (1992). *An invitation to reflexive sociology.* University of Chicago Press.

Brave Heart, Maria Yellow Horse. (1999a). Oyate ptayela: Rebuilding the Lakota nation through addressing historical trauma among Lakota parents. *Journal of Human Behavior in the Social Environment, 2*(1), 109–26.

Brave Heart, Maria Yellow Horse. (1999b). Gender differences in the historical trauma response among the Lakota. In Priscilla Day and Hilary Weaver (Eds.), *Health and the American Indian.* The Haworth Press.

Brave Heart, Maria Yellow Horse. (2004). The historical trauma response among natives and its relationship to substance abuse: A Lakota illustration. In Ethan Nebelkopf and Mary Phillips Healing (Eds.), *Health for Native Americans: Speaking in red.* Altamira Press.

Brave Heart, Maria Yellow Horse. (2014). Wakiksuyapi: Carrying the historical trauma of the Lakota. *Tulane Studies in Social Welfare, 21*, 245–66.

Brave Heart, Maria Yellow Horse and DeBruyn, Lemyra. (1998). The American Indian holocaust: Healing historical unresolved grief. *American Indian and Alaska Native Mental Health Research, 8*(2), 56–78.

Brink, S., & Zeesman, A. (1997). *Measuring social well-being: An index of social health for Canada* (Research Paper R-97-9E). Human Resources Development Canada.

Brown, D. (2002). Carrier Sekani self-government in context: Land and resources. *Western Geography, 12*, 21–67.

Browne, A., Smye, V., & Varcoe, C. (2005). The relevance of postcolonial theoretical perspectives to research in Aboriginal health. *Canadian Journal of Nursing Research, 37*(4), 16–37.

Brundtland Commission. World Commission on Environment and Development. (1987). *Our common future*. Oxford University Press.

Bryce, P.H. (1907). *Report on the Indian schools of Manitoba and the North-West Territories*. Government Printing Bureau.

Bryce, P.H. (1922). *The story of a national crime: An appeal for justice to the Indians of Canada*. James Hope & Sons.

Bud, R. (2014). "Applied science" in nineteenth-century Britain: Public discourse and the creation of meaning, 1817–1876. *History and Technology, 30*(1–2).

Cajete, G. (2000). *Native science: Natural laws of interdependence*. Clear Light Publishers.

Cajete, G. (2004). Philosophy of native science. In A. Waters (Ed.), *American Indian thought: Philosophical essays*. Blackwell Publishing.

Canadian Council on Learning. (2007). *Redefining how success is measured in First Nations, Inuit, and Métis*. Canadian Council on Learning. Retrieved from www.ccl-cca.ca

Canadian Constitution Act. (1982). Section 35: Rights of the Aboriginal Peoples of Canada. Retrieved from https://laws-lois.justice.gc.ca/eng/const/page-13.html

Candland, C. (2000). Faith as social capital: Religion and community development in southern Asia. *Policy Sciences, 33*, 355–74.

Cardinal, H. (1999). *The unjust society: The tragedy of Canada's Indians*. Douglas & McIntyre.

Carli, V. (2012). The city as a "space of opportunity": Urban Indigenous experiences and community safety partnerships. In D. Newhouse, K. FitzMaurice, T. McGuire-Adams, & D. Jette (Eds.), *Well-being in the urban Aboriginal community* (pp. 1–21). Thompson Books.

Carroll, W.K. (2004). *Critical strategies for social research*. Canadian Scholars' Press.

Castellano, M.B. (2004). Ethics of Aboriginal research. *Journal of Aboriginal Health, 1*(1), 98–114.

Castellano, M.B. (2006). *A healing journey: Reclaiming wellness. Final Report of the Aboriginal Healing Foundation* (Vol. I). Aboriginal Healing Foundation.

Castellano, M.B. & Archibald, L. (2007). Healing historic trauma: A report from the Aboriginal Healing Foundation. In J. White, S. Wingert, D. Beavon, & P. Maxim (Eds.), *Aboriginal policy research: Moving forward, making a difference* (Vol. IV). Thompson Educational Publishing.

CBC. (n.d.). *Beyond 94: Truth and reconciliation in Canada*. Retrieved from https://newsinteractives.cbc.ca/longform-single/beyond-94?&cta=1

Chandler, M.J., & Lalonde, C.E. (1998). Cultural continuity as a hedge against suicide in Canada's First Nations. *Transcultural Psychiatry, 35,* 191–219.

Chataway, C. (2002). Successful development in Aboriginal communities: Does it depend on a particular process? *The Journal of Aboriginal Economic Development, 3*(1), 76–88.

Chester, B., Robin, R., Koss, M.P., Lopez, J., & Goldman, D. (1994). Grandmother dishonored: Violence against women by male partners in American Indian communities. *Violence and Victims, 9*(3), 249–58.

Chretien, A. (2010). *A resource guide to Aboriginal well-being in Canada.* Nuclear Waste Management Organization.

Clarkson, L., Morrisette, V., & Regallet, G. (1992). *Our responsibility to the seventh generation: Indigenous peoples and sustainable development.* International Institute for Sustainable Development.

Clatworthy, S. (2008). Housing need and residential mobility among urban Aboriginal children and youth. *Horizons, 10*(1), 91–6.

Clatworthy, S.J., and Norris, M.J. (2007). Aboriginal mobility and migration in Canada: Trends, recent patterns and implications, 1971 to 2001. In J. White, S. Wingert, D. Beavon, & P. Maxim (Eds.), *Aboriginal policy research: Moving forward, making a difference* (Vol. IV). Thompson Educational Publishing.

Cloutier, E., & Langlet, E. (2014). *Aboriginal Peoples' Survey, 2012: Concepts and methods guide.* (Catalogue no. 89-653-X-No.002). Statistics Canada.

Coburn, E. (Ed.). (2015). *More will sing their way to freedom: Indigenous resistance and resurgence.* Fernwood Publishing.

Cooke, M. (2005). *The First Nations Community Well-Being Index (CWB): A conceptual review.* Strategic Research and Analysis Directorate Indian and Northern Affairs Canada.

Cooke, M. (2009). Taking a life course perspective in Indigenous research. *Canadian Issues, Journeys of a Generation: Broadening the Indigenous Well-being Policy Research Agenda,* Winter.

Cooke, M., Beavon, D., & McHardy, M. (2004). *Measuring the well-being of Aboriginal People: An application of the United Nations Human Development Index to Registered Indians in Canada, 1981–2001.* Report for the Strategic Research and Analysis Directorate, Indian and Northern Affairs Canada. Canadian Electronic Library/desLibris.

Cooke, M., Guimond, E., & McWhirter, J. (2008). The changing well-being of older registered Indians: An application of the Registered Indian Human Development Index. *Canadian Journal on Aging, 27*(4), 385–98.

Cooke, M., Mitrou, F., Lawrence, D., Guimond, E., & Beavon, D. (2007). Aboriginal well-being in four countries: An application of the UNDP's Human Development Index to Aboriginal peoples in Australia, Canada, New Zealand, and the United States. In J. White, D. Beavon, & N. Spence (Eds.), *Aboriginal well-being: Canada's continuing challenge* (pp. 87–105). Thompson Educational Publishing.

Cornell, S., & Kalt, J.P. (1998). *Sovereignty and nation-building: The development challenge in Indian country today*. Malcolm Wiener Center for Social Policy.

Corntassel, J. (2008). Toward sustainable self determination: Rethinking the contemporary Indigenous-rights discourse. *Alternatives. 33*(1), 105–32. https://doi.org/10.1177/030437540803300106

Corntassel, J. (2012). Re-envisioning resurgence: Indigenous pathways to decolonization and sustainable self-determination. *Decolonization: Indigeneity, Education & Society 1*(1), 86–101.

Corntassel, J., Chaw-win-is, & T'lakwadzi. (2009). Indigenous storytelling, truth-telling, and community approaches to reconciliation. *English Studies in Canada, 35*(1), 137–59.

Corntassel, J., & Bryce, C. (2012). Practicing sustainable self-determination: Indigenous approaches to cultural restoration and revitalization. *Brown Journal of World Affairs, 18*(2), 151–62.

Corntassel, J., & Scow, M. (2017). Everyday acts of resurgence: Indigenous approaches to everydayness in fatherhood. *New Diversities, 19*(2), 55–68. Retrieved from https://newdiversities.mmg.mpg.de/?page_id=3194

Côté, R. (2012). Networks of advantage: Urban Indigenous entrepreneurship and the importance of social capital. In D. Newhouse, K. FitzMaurice, T. McGuire-Adams, & D. Jetté (Eds.), *Well-being in the urban Aboriginal community – fostering Biimaadiziwin*. Thompson Educational Publishing.

Coulthard, G. (2014). *Red skin, white masks: Rejecting the colonial politics of recognition*. University of Minnesota Press.

Cox, L. & Nilsen, A.G. (2014). *We make our own history: Marxism and social movements in the twilight of neoliberalism*. Pluto Press.

Crossley, N. (2003). From reproduction to transformation: Social movement fields and the radical habitus. *Theory, Culture & Society, 20*(6), 43–68.

Cummins, R., Woerner, J., Gibson, A., Lai, L., Weinberg, M., & Collard, J. (2008). *Australian unity wellbeing index survey 19*. The School of Psychology and The Australian Centre on Quality of Life, Deakin University, and Australian Unity Limited.

Daly, H. (2009). *The (un)happy planet index*. The New Economics Foundation. Retrieved from https://static1.squarespace.com/static/5735c421e32140 2778ee0ce9/t/578de9f729687f525e004f7b/1468918272070/2009+Happy +Planet+Index+report.pdf

Darnovsky, M., Epstein, B.L., & Flacks, R. (1995). *Cultural politics and social movements*. Temple University Press.

Daschuk, J. (2013). *Clearing the plains: Disease, politics of starvation and the loss of Aboriginal life*. University of Regina Press.

Deer, Cecile. (2012). Reflexivity. In M. Grenfell (Ed.), *Pierre Bourdieu: Key concepts* (2nd ed., pp. 195–208). Acumen Publishing Limited.

Deer, F., & Falconberg, T. (2016). *Indigenous perspectives on education for well-being in Canada*. Education for Sustainable Well-Being Press.

Deloria, V., Jr., & Wildcat, D.R (2001). *Power and place: Indian education in America*. Fulcrum Publishing.

Denis, J.S. (2015). A four directions model: Understanding the rise and resonance of an Indigenous self-determination movement. In E. Coburn (Ed.), *More will sing their way to freedom: Indigenous resistance and resurgence* (pp. 208–28). Fernwood Publishing.

Denzin, N., Lincoln, Y., & Smith, L. (2008). *Handbook of critical and Indigenous methodologies*. Sage Publications.

Dickson, G. (2000). Aboriginal grandmother's experience with health promotion and participatory action research. *Qualitative Health Research, 10*(2), 188–213.

Drabsch, T. (2012, July). *Measuring wellbeing* [Briefing paper no 4]. NSW Parliamentary Research Service, Parliament of New South Wales, Australia. Retrieved from https://www.parliament.nsw.gov.au /researchpapers/Documents/measuring-wellbeing/Wellbeing.pdf

Environics Institute. (2010). *Urban Aboriginal peoples study*. Environics Institute.

Eriksson, M., & Lindstrom, B. (2008). A salutogenic interpretation of the Ottawa Charter. *Health Promotion International, 23*(2), 190–9.

Feagin, J.R. (2004). Social justice and sociology: Agendas for the twenty-first century. In W. Carroll (Ed.), *Critical strategies for social research* (pp. 29–43). Canadian Scholars' Press.

Felligi, I. (1996). *Strengthening our policy capacity*. Report of the Deputy Ministers' Task Force. Canadian Centre for Management Development.

First Nations Health Authority. (n.d.). *Relationship agreement*. Retrieved from http://www.fnha.ca/Documents/FNHC_FNHA_FNHDA_Relationship _Agreement.pdf

First Nations Health Authority. (2011, May 24–26). *Summary report*. Gathering Wisdom for a Shared Journey IV, Richmond, British Columbia. Retrieved from https://gathering-wisdom.ca/wp-content/uploads/2019/10 /Gathering_Wisdom_IV_Summary_Report.pdf

First Nations Health Authority. (2012a, May 15–17). *Summary report*. Gathering Wisdom V for a Shared Journey. Retrieved from https://gathering-wisdom .ca/wp-content/uploads/2019/10/Gathering_Wisdom_V_Summary _Report.pdf

First Nations Health Authority. (2012b). *Together in wellness: A report on the progress of the integration and the improvement of health services for First Nations in British Columbia*. Tripartite Committee on First Nations Health Interim Annual Report 2011/2012. Retrieved from http://www.health.gov.bc.ca /library/publications/year/2012/together-in-wellness.pdf

First Nations Health Authority (2013a). *Annual report: 2012–2013*. Retrieved from http://www.fnha.ca/Documents/FNHA_Annual_Report_2012-13.pdf

First Nations Health Authority. (2013b, April 16). *Community health and wellness indicators*. Health Indicators Strategy Table, Health Knowledge and Information Health Actions.

First Nations Health Authority, (2016a). *Governance and accountability*. Retrieved from http://www.fnha.ca/about/governance-and-accountability

First Nations Health Authority. (2016b). *FNHA board of directors*. Retrieved from http://www.fnha.ca/about/governance-and-accountability/fnha -board-of-directors

First Nations Health Authority. (2016c). *About the FNHA*. Retrieved from https://www.fnha.ca/about

First Nations Health Authority. (2016d). *First Nations perspective on health and wellness*. Retrieved from http://www.fnha.ca/wellness/wellness -and-the-first-nations-health-authority/first-nations-perspective-on -wellness

First Nations Health Authority. (2016e). *Annual report: 2015–2016*. Retrieved from https://www.fnha.ca/about/news-and-events/news/2015-16-first -nations-health-authority-annual-report

First Nations Health Council. (2011). *Implementing the vision: BC First Nations health governance*. First Nations Health Authority. Retrieved from https:// www.fnha.ca/Documents/FNHC_Health_Governance_Book.pdf

First Nations Health Council. (2016, November 30–December 2). *Summary report*. Gathering Wisdom for a Shared Journey VIII. Retrieved from https://gathering-wisdom.ca/wp-content/uploads/2019/10/Gathering -Wisdom-for-a-Shared-Journey-VIII-Summary-Report_WEB.pdf

First Nations Information Governance Centre. (2012). *First Nations Regional Health Survey (RHS) 2008/10: National Report on Adults, Youth and Children living in First Nations Communities*. Ottawa: First Nations Centre. Retrieved December 30, 2016 from http://fnigc.ca/sites/default/files/docs/first _nations_regional_health_survey_rhs_2008-10_-_national_report.pdf

Fiske, J., Newell, M., & George, E. (2001). *First Nations women and governance: A study of custom and innovation among Lake Babine Nation women*. Status of Women Canada.

Flaherty, J.M. (2012). *Jobs, growth and long-term prosperity: Economic Action Plan 2012*. Public Works and Government Services Canada.

Fleras, A., and Elliott, J.L. (1996). *Unequal relations: An introduction to race, ethnic and Aboriginal dynamics in Canada*. Prentice Hall Canada.

Foster, L., & Keller, C.P. (2011). Wellness frameworks and indicators: An update. In *The British Columbia Atlas of Wellness, Western Geographical Series*, (Chapter 2, Volume 42). Western Geographical Press. https://dspace .library.uvic.ca/handle/1828/3838

Foucault, M. (1972). *Power/knowledge: Selected interviews and other writings 1972–1977* (C. Gordon, Ed.). Pantheon.

Frideres, J. (2010). Building bridges: Immigrant, visible minority, and Aboriginal families in the twenty-first century. In D. Cheal (Ed.), *Canadian families today: New perspectives* (2nd ed., pp. 183–99). Oxford University Press.

Frideres, J., & Gadacz, R. (2006). *Aboriginal peoples in Canada* (7th ed.). Prentice Hall.

Gagné, M.A. (1998). The role of dependency and colonialism in generating trauma in First Nations citizens: The James Bay Cree. In Y. Danieli (Ed.), *International handbook of multigenerational legacies of trauma* (pp. 355–71). Plenum Press.

Gehl, Lynn. (n.d.) *Ally bill of responsibilities*. Retrieved from https://www.lynngehl.com/ally-bill-of-responsibilities.html

Goldman, R., & Tickameyer, A. (1984). Status attainment and commodity form: Stratification in historical perspective. *American Sociological Review, 49*(2), 196–209.

Gone, J.P. (2011). The red road to wellness: Cultural reclamation in a Native First Nation community treatment center. *American Journal of Community Psychology, 47*(1–2), 187–202.

Gone, J.P. (2013). Redressing First Nations historical trauma: Theorizing mechanisms for Indigenous culture as mental health treatment. *Transcultural Psychiatry, 50*(5), 683–706. https://doi.org/10.1177/1363461513487669

Gone, J.P., & Kirmayer, L.J. (2010). On the wisdom of considering culture and context in psychopathology. In T. Millon, R.F. Krueger, & E. Simonsen (Eds.), *Contemporary directions in psychopathology: Scientific foundations of the DSM-V and ICD-11* (pp. 72–96). Guilford.

Gone, J.P., Kirmayer, L.J., & Moses, J. (2014). Rethinking historical trauma. *Transcultural Psychiatry 51*(3).

Government of British Columbia. (n.d). *The transformative change accord: First Nations health plan supporting the health and wellness of First Nations in British Columbia*. Retrieved from http://www.health.gov.bc.ca/library/publications/year/2006/first_nations_health_implementation_plan.pdf

Gracey, M., & King, M. (2009). Indigenous health part 1: Determinants and disease patterns. *Lancet, 374*(9683), 65–75.

Gray, M., Coates, J., & Yellow Bird, M. (2008). *Indigenous social work around the world: Towards culturally relevant education and practice*. Ashgate.

Guimond, E., Fonda, M., and Jetté, D. (2012). *Aboriginal populations in Canadian cities: Why are they growing so fast?* The Strategic Research Directorate Research Brief series. Aboriginal Affairs and Northern Development Canada.

Haig-Brown, C. (1992). Choosing border work. *Canadian Journal of Native Education, 19*(1), 96–116.

References

131

Hallett, D., Chandler, M.J., & Lalonde, C.E. (2007). Aboriginal language knowledge and youth suicide. *Cognitive Development, 22*(3), 392–9.

Harris, Cole. (2003). *Making native space: Colonialism, resistance, and reserves in British Columbia.* UBC Press.

Haque, S.M. (2004). The myths of economic growth (GNP): Implications for human development. In G. Mudacumura and M. Haque (Eds.), *Handbook of development policy studies* (pp. 1–24). Marcel Dekker.

Hawthorn, H. (Ed.). (1967). *A survey of the contemporary Indians of Canada: Economic, political, educational needs and policies.* Queen's Printer Press. Retrieved from http://caid.ca/HawRep1a1966.pdf

Health Canada. (2011). *British Columbia tripartite framework agreement on First Nations health governance.* Retrieved from https://www.sac-isc.gc.ca/eng/1584706392620/1584706415366

Health Canada. (2002). *A new approach to Aboriginal health.* Commission on the Future of Health Care in Canada: Final Report. Retrieved from http://publications.gc.ca/collections/Collection/CP32-85-2002E.pdf

HealthlinkBC. (2015). *Aboriginal/First Nations health.* Retrieved from https://www.healthlinkbc.ca/health-topics/common-health-concerns/first-nations Last accessed December 2016.

Heck, R.H., & Thomas, S.L. (2015). *An introduction to multilevel modeling techniques: MLM and SEM approaches using Mplus* (3rd ed.). Routledge.

Helin, C. (2006). *Dances with dependency: Indigenous success through self-reliance.* Orca Spirit Publishing & Communications.

Helliwell, J.F. (2001). Social capital, the economy and well-being. In K.G. Banting (Ed.), *The review of economic performance and social progress* (pp. 43–60). The Institute for Research on Public Policy.

Helliwell, J.F., & McKitrick, R. (1999). Comparing capital mobility across provincial and national borders. *Canadian Journal of Economics, 32*(5), 1164–73.

Hewitt, T. (2016, January 25). *Canada's researchers eager to support truth and reconciliation efforts.* University Affairs. Retrieved from http://www.universityaffairs.ca/opinion/in-my-opinion/canadas-researchers-eager-to-support-truth-and-reconciliation-efforts/

Hill, G., & Cooke, M. (2014). How do you build a community? Developing community capacity and social capital in an urban Aboriginal setting. *Pimatisiwin, 11*(3), 421–32.

Hodge, F., Pasqua, A., Marquez, C., & Geishirt-Cantrell, B. (2011). Utilizing traditional storytelling to promote wellness in American Indian communities. *Journal of Transcultural Nursing, 13*(1), 6–11.

Hull, J. (2006). *Aboriginal women: A profile from the 2001 Census.* Women's Issues and Gender Equality Directorate Indian and Northern Affairs Canada.

Hunt, S., & Holmes, C. (2015). Everyday decolonization: Living a decolonizing queer politics. *Journal of Lesbian Studies, 19*(2), 154–72. https://doi.org /10.1080/10894160.2015.970975

Hutchinson, P. (2006). An exploratory analysis of linkage social capital as a determinant of health. *Pimatisiwin 4*(1), 105–18

INAC. (2015a). *Community well-being index.* Indigenous Affairs and Northern Development (formerly AANDC). Retrieved from https://www.aadnc -aandc.gc.ca/eng/1100100016579/1100100016580

INAC. (2015b). *Urban Indigenous peoples.* Indigenous Affairs and Northern Development (formerly AANDC). Retrieved from https://www.aadnc -aandc.gc.ca/eng/1100100014265/1369225120949

INAC. (2016). *Recognized Indian residential schools.* Retrieved December 30, 2016 from https://www.aadnc-aandc.gc.ca/eng/1100100015606/1100100015611

Indigenous Action. (2014). *Accomplices not allies: Abolishing the ally industrial complex.* Retrieved from https://www.indigenousaction.org/accomplices -not-allies-abolishing-the-ally-industrial-complex/

Institute of Urban Studies in collaboration with Assembly of Manitoba Chiefs, Manitoba Métis Federation. (2004). *First Nations/Métis/Inuit mobility study. Final report.* Institute of Urban Studies, The University of Winnipeg.

Iwama, M., Marshall, M., Marshall, A., & Bartlett, C. (2009). Two-eyed seeing and the language of healing in community-based research. *Canadian Journal of Native Education, 32*(2), 3–23.

Kelley M.L., Habian, S., & Prince, H. (2012). Caregiving for Elders in First Nations communites: Social system perspective on barriers and challenges. *Canadian Journal on Aging, 31*(2), 209–22. Cambridge University Press.

Kelm, M. (1998). *Colonizing bodies: Aboriginal health and healing in British Columbia, 1900–50.* UBC Press.

Kenny, C. (2002). *North American Indian, Métis and Inuit women speak about culture, education and work.* Status of Women Canada.

Kim, D., Subramanian, S.V., & Kawachi, I. (2006). Bonding versus bridging social capital and their association with self-rated health: A multilevel analysis of 40 US communities. *Journal of Epidemiological Community Health, 60*(2), 116–22.

Kirmayer, L.J., Dandeneau, S., Marshall, E., Phillips, M.K., & Williamson, K.J. (2011). Rethinking resilience from Indigenous perspectives. *Canadian Journal of Psychiatry, 56*(2), 84–91.

Kirmayer, L.J., Dandeneau, S., Marshall, E., Phillips, M.K., & Williamson, K.J. (2012). Toward an ecology of stories: Indigenous perspectives on resilience. In M. Ungar (Ed.), *The social ecology of resilience* (pp. 399–414). Springer.

Kirmayer, L.J., Simpson, C., & Cargo, M. (2003). Healing traditions: Culture, community and mental health promotion with Canadian Aboriginal peoples. *Australasian Psychiatry, 11*(suppl 1), S15–S23.

Knibb-Lamouche, J. (2012, November 14). *Leveraging culture to address health inequalities: Examples from Native communities: Workshop summary.* Commissioned paper prepared for the Institute on Medicine. Roundtable on the Promotion of Health Equity and the Elimination of Health Disparities, Seattle, Washington.

Kovach, M. (2005). Emerging from the margins: Indigenous methodologies. In S. Strega and L. Brown (Eds.), *Research as resistance: Critical, Indigenous and anti-oppressive approaches* (pp. 19–36). Canadian Scholars' Press.

Kovach, M. (2009). *Indigenous methodologies: Characteristics, conversations, and context.* University of Toronto Press.

Kral, M. (2012). Postcolonial suicide among Inuit in Arctic Canada. *Culture, Medicine and Psychiatry, 36*(2), 306–25.

Laliberte, N. (2012). *Indigenous Health Indicator Frameworks report.* Prepared for the Tripartite Health Indicators Planning Committee. Internal working document of the First Nations Health Authority.

Lavoie, J., O'Neal, J., Reading J., & Allard, Y. (2008). Community healing & Aboriginal self-government. In Y. Belanger (Ed.), *Aboriginal self-government in Canada: Current trends & issues* (3rd ed., pp. 173–205). Purich Publishing.

Lawson-Te Aho, K., & Liu, J.H. (2010). Indigenous suicide and colonization: The legacy of violence and the necessity of self-determination. *International Journal of Conflict and Violence, 4*(1), 124–133.

Ledogar, R.J., & Fleming, J. (2008a). Social capital and resilience: A review of concepts and selected literature relevant to Aboriginal youth resilience research. *Pimatisiwin, 6*(2), 25–46.

Ledogar, R.J., & Fleming, J. (2008b). Resilience, an evolving concept: A review of literature relevant to Aboriginal research. *Pimatisiwin, 6*(2), 7–23.

Ledogar, R.J., & Fleming, J. (2008c). Resilience and Indigenous spirituality: A literature review. *Pimatisiwin, 6*(2), 47–64.

Levitte, Y. (2004). Bonding social capital in entrepreneurial developing communities: Survival networks or barriers? *Journal of the Community Development Society, 35*, 44–64.

Lindstrom, B., & Eriksson, M. (2009). The salutogenic approach to the making of HiAP/healthy public policy: Illustrated by a case study. *Global Health Promotion, 16*(1), 17–28.

Linklater, R. (2014). *Decolonizing trauma work: Indigenous stories and strategies.* Fernwood Publishing.

Lofors, J., & Sundquist, K. (2007). Low-linking social capital as a predictor of mental disorders: A cohort study of 4.5 million Swedes. *Social Science & Medicine, 64*(1), 21–34.

Loppie-Reading, C., & Wien, F. (2009). *Health inequalities and the social determinants of Aboriginal peoples health.* National Collaborating Centre for Aboriginal Health.

Marx, K. (1978). *The Marx-Engels reader* (Robert C. Tucker, Ed.). W. W. Norton and Co.

Maté, G. (2008). *In the realm of hungry ghosts: Close encounters with addictions.* Alfred Knopf.

Maxim, P., White, J., & Beavon, D. (2003). Dispersion and polarization of income among Aboriginal and non-Aboriginal Canadians. In J. White, P. Maxim, & D. Beavon (Eds.), *Aboriginal conditions: Research as a foundation for public policy* (pp. 222–47). UBC Press.

McCaslin, W., & Boyer, Y. (2009). First Nations communities at risk and in crisis: Justice and security. *Journal of Aboriginal Health, 5*(2).

McGillivray, M. (1991). The human development index: Yet another redundant composite development indicator? *World Development, 19*(10), 1461–8.

McHardy, M., & O'Sullivan, E. (2004). *First Nations community well-being in Canada: The Community Well-Being Index (CWB) 2001.* Strategic Research and Analysis.

Menzies, C. (2001). Reflections on research with, for, and among Indigenous peoples. *Canadian Journal of Native Education, 25*(1), 19–36.

Mignone, J. (2003). *Social capital in First Nations communities: Conceptual development and instrument validation* [Unpublished doctoral dissertation]. University of Manitoba.

Mignone, J. (2009). Social capital and Aboriginal communities: A critical assessment, synthesis and assessment of the body of knowledge on social capital with emphasis on Aboriginal communities. *Journal de la santé autochtone, 5*(3), 100–47.

Mignone, J., & O'Neil, J. (2005a). Social capital and youth suicide risk factors in First Nations communities. *Canadian Journal of Public Health, 96*(Suppl 1), S51–S54.

Mignone J., & O'Neil, J. (2005b). Social capital as a health determinant in First Nations: An exploratory study in three communities. *Journal of Aboriginal Health, 2*(1), 26–33.

Miller, J.R. (1991). *Skyscrapers hide the heavens – a history of Indian–white relations in Canada.* University of Toronto Press.

Million, Dian. (2013). *Therapeutic nations: Healing in an age of Indigenous human rights.* The University of Arizona Press

Milloy, J.S. (1999). A national crime: The Canadian government and the residential school system, 1879 to 1986. In S. Fournier & E. Crey (Eds.), *Stolen from our embrace* (pp. 91–2). Douglas & McIntyre.

Monchalin, L. (2016). *The colonial problem: An Indigenous perspective on crime and injustice in Canada.* University of Toronto Press.

Moore, R. (2012). Capital. In M. Grenfell (Ed.), *Pierre Bourdieu: Key concepts* (2nd ed., pp. 98–113). Grenfell Acumen Publishing Limited.

Moore, S., Shiell, A., Hawe, P., & Haines, V.A. (2005). The privileging of communitarian ideas: Citation practices and translation of social capital into public health research. *American Journal of Public Health 95*(8), 1330–7.

Morrisette, P.J. (1994). The holocaust of First Nation People: Residual effects on parenting and treatment implications. *Contemporary Family Therapy, 16*(5), 381–92.

Mosby, I, (2013). Administering colonial science: Nutrition research and human biomedical experimentation in Aboriginal communities and residential schools, 1942–1952. *Social History, 46*(91), 145–72.

Mundel, E., & Chapman, G.E. (2010). A decolonizing approach to health promotion in Canada: The case of the urban Aboriginal community kitchen garden project. *Health Promotion International, 25*(2), 166–73.

National Association of Friendship Centres. (2016). *Urban programming for Indigenous peoples.* Retrieved on December 30, 2016 from http://nafc.ca/en/national-programs/community-capacity-supports/; see also https://www.nafc.ca/en/programs-initiatives/urban-programming-for-indigenous-peoples

Nettelbeck, A. (2016). "We are sure of your sympathy": Aboriginal uses of the politics of protection in nineteenth-century Australia and Canada. *Journal of Colonialism and Colonial History, 17*(1), 1–21.

Neu, D., and Therrien, R. (2003) *Accounting for genocide: Canada's bureaucratic assault on Aboriginal people.* Fernwood Publishing.

Newhouse, D., and Fitzmaurice, K. (2012). Introduction. In D. Newhouse, K. FitzMaurice, T. McGuire-Adams, & D. Jetté (Eds.), *Well-being in the Aboriginal community: Fostering Biimaadiziwin, a national research conference on urban Aboriginal Peoples* (pp. ix–xxi). Thompson Educational Publishing.

Newhouse, D., & McGuire-Adams, T. (2012). Preface. In D. Newhouse, K. FitzMaurice, T. McGuire-Adams, & D. Jetté (Eds.), *Well-being in the Aboriginal community: Fostering Biimaadiziwin, a national research conference on urban Aboriginal peoples* (pp. vii–viii). Thompson Educational Publishing.

Norris, D., & Siggner, A. (2003). *What Census and the Aboriginal Peoples Survey tell us about Aboriginal conditions in Canada.* Paper presented at the Aboriginal Strategies Conference, Edmonton.

Norris, M. (2006). Aboriginal languages in Canada: Trends and perspectives on maintenance and revitalization. In J.P. White, S. Wingert, D. Beavan, & P. Maxim (Eds.), *Aboriginal policy research: Moving forward, making a difference* (Vol. 3, pp. 197–226). Thompson Educational Publishing.

Norris, M., & Clatworthy, S. (2003). Aboriginal mobility and migration within urban Canada: Outcomes, factors and implications. In D. Newhouse and E. Peters (Eds.), *Not strangers in these parts | Urban Aboriginal peoples* (pp. 51–78). Policy Research Initiative.

Norris, M., & Clatworthy, S. (2011). Urbanization and migration patterns of Aboriginal populations in Canada: A half century in review. *Aboriginal Policy Studies, 1*(1), 13–77.

Northern Gateway. (2016). *Building a better project: A letter to communities.* Retrieved on December 29, 2016 from http://www.gatewayfacts.ca /Benefits/Jobs-And-Training.aspx

O'Brien, D.J., Phillips, J.L., & Patsiorkovsky, V.V. (2005). Linking Indigenous bonding and bridging social capital. *Regional Studies, 39*(8), 1041–51.

OECD. (2000). *Measuring well-being and progress: Well-being research.* Retrieved from http://www.oecd.org/document/33/0,3746,en_2649_33715_47835039 _1_1_1_1,00.html

Olsen, W. (2012). *Data collection: Key debates and methods in social research.* Sage Publications.

O'Sullivan, E. (2006). *The Community Well-Being (CWB) Index: Well-being in First Nations communities, 1981–2001 and into the future.* Indian Affairs and Northern Development, Strategic Analysis Directorate.

O'Sullivan, E. (2010). *Aboriginal language use and socioeconomic wellbeing: A multilevel analysis* [Unpublished doctoral dissertation]. McMaster University.

O'Sullivan, E., & McHardy, M. (2007). The Community Well-being Index (CWB): Well-being in First Nations communities, present, past, & future. In J. White, D. Beavon, & N. Spence (Eds.), *Aboriginal well-being: Canada's continuing challenge* (pp. 111–40). Thompson Educational Publishing.

Palmater, P. (2017). Death by poverty: The lethal impacts of colonialism. In W. Antony, J. Antony, & L. Samuelson (Eds.), *Power and resistance: Critical thinking about Canadian social issues* (6th ed., pp. 51–81). Fernwood Publishing.

Peters, E. (2009). Urban Aboriginal Economic Development Network website. Retrieved April 14, 2017 from abdc.bc.ca/uaed/

Peters E., and Anderson, C. (2013). *Indigenous in the city: Contemporary identities and cultural innovation.* UBC Press.

Peters, E., Clatworthy, S., & Norris, M.J. (2013). The urbanization of Aboriginal populations in Canada: A half century in review. In E. Peters & C. Andersen (Eds.), *Indigenous in the city: Contemporary identities and cultural innovation* (pp. 29–45). UBC Press.

Portes, A. (1998). Social capital: Its origins and applications in contemporary sociology. *Annual Review of Sociology, 24,* 1–24.

Portes, A., & Landolt, P. (1996). The downside of social capital. *The American Prospect, 26,* 18–23.

Portes, A., & Landolt. P. (2000). Social capital: Promise and pitfalls of its role in development. *Journal of Latin American Studies, 32*(2), 529–47.

Putnam, R.D. (1993). *Making democracy work: Civic traditions in modern Italy.* Princeton University Press.

Putnam, R.D. (1995). Tuning in, tuning out: The strange disappearance of social capital in America. *Political Science and Politics, 28*(4), 664–83.

Puxley, C. (2015, May 31). How many First Nations kids died in residential schools? Justice Murray Sinclair says Canada needs answers. *The Star.* Retrieved from https://www.thestar.com/news/canada/2015/05/31/how-many-first-nations-kids-died-in-residential-schools-justice-murray-sinclair-says-canada-needs-answers.html

Quinless, J. (2009). *Urban Aboriginal population: A statistical profile of Aboriginal people residing in the city of Edmonton in 2006.* Prepared for the Aboriginal Relations Office and the Office of the Deputy Manager, City of Edmonton.

Quinless, J. (2014). Family matters: Household size in relation to the well-being of Aboriginal school-aged children living off reserve. *Journal of Aboriginal Policy Studies, 3*(1/2), 5–28.

Quinless, J. (2015). Indigenous well-being in Canada: Understanding wellness in the context of knowledge networks, interconnectedness and social change. *The Global Studies Journal, 8*(3).

Quinless, J. (2017). *Decolonizing bodies: A First Nations perspective on the determinants of urban Indigenous health and wellness in Canada* [Unpublished doctoral dissertation]. University of Victoria.

Quinless, J., & Corntassel, J. (2018, March 9). *Responsive research in an era of reconciliation.* IPAC, Vancouver.

Quinless, J., & Manmohan, R. (2015). Families in transition: The impact of family relationships and work on mobility patterns of Aboriginal people living in urban centres across Canada. *Aboriginal Policy Studies, 5*(2), 113–35.

Reading, J., Kmetic, A., & Gideon, V. (2007). *First Nations holistic policy and planning model.* Discussion paper for the World Health Organization Commission on Social Determinants of Health. Retrieved from http://ahrnets.ca/files/2011/02/AFN_Paper_2007.pdf

Regan, P. (2010). *Unsettling the settler within, Indian residential schools, truth telling, and reconciliation in Canada.* UBC Press.

Richmond, C., Ross, N.A., & Egeland, G.M. (2007) Societal resources and thriving health: A new approach for understanding the health of Indigenous Canadians. *American Journal of Public Health, 97*(10), 1827–33.

Ritchie, J., Lewis, J., Nicholls, C.M., Ormston, R. (2014). *Qualitative research practice: A guide for social science students and researchers.* Sage Publications.

Robson, K., & Sanders, C. (Eds.). (2009). *Quantifying theory: Pierre Bourdieu.* Springer Science + Business Media B.V.

Rogers, S., DeGagné, M., & Dewar, J. (2012). *Speaking my truth: Reflections on reconciliation & residential school.* Aboriginal Healing Foundation.

Ross, R. (1996). *Returning to the teachings: Exploring Aboriginal justice.* Penguin Canada.

Royal Commission on Aboriginal People. (1996a). *Report of the Royal Commission on Aboriginal Peoples. Volume 1: Looking forward, looking back.* Canada Communication Group. Retrieved from http://data2.archives.ca/e/e448/e011188230-01.pdf

Royal Commission on Aboriginal Peoples. (1996b). *Report of the Royal Commission on Aboriginal Peoples. Volume 5: Renewal: A twenty-year commitment.* Minister of Supply and Services. Retrieved from https://qspace.library.queensu.ca/bitstream/handle/1974/6874/RRCAP5_combined.pdf?sequence=1&isAllowed=y

Salée, D. with the assistance of D. Newhouse and C. Lévesque. (2006). Quality of life of Aboriginal people in Canada: An analysis of current research. *IRPP Choices, 12*(6), 1–38.

Sayer, J., MacDonald, K., Fiske, J., Newell, M., George, E., & Cornet, W. (2001). *First Nations women, governance and the Indian Act: A collection of policy research reports.* Research Directorate, Status of Women Canada. Retrieved from https://fngovernance.org/wp-content/uploads/2020/07/First_Nation_Women_and_Governance.pdf

Scott, D.C. (1920). *The Indian problem.* National Archives of Canada, Record Group 10, volume 6810, file 470-2-3, volume 7, pp. 55 (L-3) and 63 (N-3).

Sellars, Bev. (2013). *They called me number one: Secrets and survival at an Indian residential school.* Vancouver: Talonbooks.

Silver, J., Ghorayshi, P., Hay, J., & Klyne, D. (2006). *In a voice of their own: Urban Aboriginal community development.* Canadian Centre for Policy Alternatives. Retrieved from http://www.policyalternatives.ca/sites/default/files/uploads/publications/Manitoba_Pubs/2006/In_A_Voice_Of_Their_Own.pdf

Simeone, T. (2007). *The Harvard Project on American Indian economic development: Findings and considerations.* Library of Parliament.

Simpson, L.R. (2004). Anticolonial strategies for the recovery and maintenance of Indigenous knowledge. *American Indian Quarterly, 28*(3&4), 373–84.

Simpson, L.B. (2011). *Dancing on our turtle's back: Stories of Nishnaabeg re-creation, resurgence and a new emergence.* Arbeiter Ring.

Simpson, L.B. (2017). *As we have always done.* University of Minnesota Press.

Smith, L.T. (1999). *Decolonizing methodologies: Research and Indigenous peoples.* Zed Books.

Smith, L.T. (2006). Colonizing knowledges. In Roger Maaka and Chris Andersen (Eds.), *The Indigenous experience: Global perspectives.* Canadian Scholars' Press.

Smith, L.T. (2012). *Decolonizing methodologies: Research and Indigenous people* (2nd ed.). Otago University Press.

Snelgrove, C., Dhamoon. R., & Corntassel, J. (2014) Unsettling settler colonialism: The discourse and politics of settlers, and solidarity with Indigenous nations. *Decolonization: Indigeneity, Education & Society, 3*(2), 1–32.

Social Sciences and Humanities Research Council. (2019). *Indigenous research statement of principles.* Retrieved from http://www.sshrc-crsh.gc.ca/about -au_sujet/policies-politiques/statements-enonces/aboriginal_research -recherche_autochtone-eng.aspx

Stake, R.E. (2005). Qualitative case studies. In N.K. Denzin and Y.S. Lincoln (Eds.), *The Sage handbook of qualitative research* (3rd ed., pp. 433–66). Sage Publications.

Starblanket, G., & Stark, H. (2018) Toward a relational paradigm: Four points for consideration: Knowledge, gender, land and modernity. In M. Asch, J. Borrows, & J. Tully (Eds.), *Resurgence and reconciliation: Indigenous-settler relations and earth teachings.* University of Toronto Press.

Statistics Canada. (2011). *The Census of Population questionnaire 2A and National Household Survey.* Statistics Canada.

Statistics Canada. (2012). *Aboriginal peoples in Canada in 2012: Inuit, Métis and First Nations.* Catalogue no. 97-558-XIE. Minister of Industry.

Statistics Canada. (2016). *Income reference guide, National Household Survey, 2011.* Catalogue no. 99-014-XWE2011006. Minister of Industry.

Stevenson, Lisa. (2014). *Life beside itself: Imagining care in the Canadian Arctic.* University of California Press.

Stiglitz, J.E., Sen, A., and Fitoussi, P. (2010). *Report by the Commission on the Measurement of Economic Performance and Social Progress.* Retrieved from http://library.bsl.org.au/jspui/bitstream/1/1267/1/Measurement_of _economic_performance_and_social_progress.pdf

Strega, S., & Brown, L. (2015). *Research as resistance: Revisiting critical, Indigenous, and anti-oppressive approaches* (2nd ed.). Canadian Scholars' Press.

The Centre for Bhutan Studies. (2008). *Gross national happiness. Explanation of GNH index.* Retrieved on December 30, 2016 from http://www .grossnationalhappiness.com/gnhIndex/intruductionGNH.aspx

Thomas, R. (2015). Qwul'sih'yah'maht: Honouring the oral traditions of my ancestors through storytelling. In S. Strega & L. Brown, (2015). *Research as resistance: Revisiting critical, Indigenous, and anti-oppressive approaches* (2nd ed., pp. 237–54). Canadian Scholars' Press.

Truth and Reconciliation Commission of Canada. (2015). *Honouring the truth and reconciling for the future. Summary report of the Truth and Reconciliation Commission of Canada: Calls to action.* James Lorimer & Company Ltd.

Truth Commission into Genocide in Canada. (2001). *Hidden from history: The Canadian holocaust. The untold story of the genocide of Aboriginal peoples by church and state in Canada.* Truth Commission into Genocide in Canada.

Tuck, E. (2009). Suspending damage: A letter to communities. *Harvard Educational Review, 79*(3), 409–27.

Tuck, E., & Yang, K.W. (2012). Decolonization is not a metaphor. *Decolonization: Indigeneity, Education & Society, 1*(1), 1–40.

United Nations Development Programme (UNDP). (1990). *Human development report 1990.* Oxford University Press.

UNDP. (2016). *Composite indices: HDI and beyond.* Retrieved from http://hdr .undp.org/en/statistics/understanding/indices

Unicef Canada. (2009). *Canadian supplement to the state of the world's children 2009: Aboriginal children's health: Leaving no child behind.* Canadian UNICEF Committee. Retrieved from https://www.nccah-ccnsa.ca/docs/child%20 and%20youth/Report%20Summary%20Leaving%20no%20child%20 behind.pdf

United Nations (n.d). *Who are Indigenous peoples?* Retrieved from http://www .un.org/esa/socdev/unpfii/documents/5session_factsheet1.pdf

United Nations (2008). *United Nations Declaration on the Rights of Indigenous Peoples.* Retrieved from http://www.un.org/esa/socdev/unpfii /documents/DRIPS_en.pdf

United Nations. Human Rights Office of the High Comissioner. (2020, May 18). *COVID-19 is devastating Indigenous communities worldwide, and it's not only about health – UN expert warns.* Retrieved from https://www.ohchr.org /EN/NewsEvents/Pages/DisplayNews.aspx?NewsID=25893&LangID=E

University Affairs. (2016). *Canada's researchers eager to support truth and reconciliation efforts.* Retrieved from http://www.universityaffairs.ca /opinion/in-my-opinion/canadas-researchers-eager-to-support-truth-and -reconciliation-efforts/

Ura, K., Alkire, S., Zangmo, T., & Wangdi, K. (2012). *A short guide to gross national happiness index.* The Centre for Bhutan Studies.

Van Uchelen, C.P., Davidson, S.F., Quressette, S.V., Brasfield, C.R., & Demeras, L.H. (1997). What makes us strong: Urban Aboriginal perspectives on wellness and strength. *Canadian Journal of Community Mental Health, 16*(2), 37–50.

Veenstra, G. (2002). Social capital and health, plus wealth, income inequality and regional health governance. *Social Science & Medicine, 54*(6), 849–68.

Veentsra, G. (2009). Transmutations of capitals in Canada: A "social space" approach. In K. Robson & C. Sanders (Eds.), *Quantifying theory: Pierre Bourdieu.* Springer Science + Business Media B.V.

Verschuren, P. (2003). Case study as a research strategy: Some ambiguities and opportunities. *International Journal of Social Research Methodology, 6*(2), 121–39.

Vizenor, G. (2007). Literary chance: Essays on Native American survivance. *First Nations Perspectives.* University of Valencia.

Walia, H. (2012), *Decolonizing together: Moving beyond a politics of solidarity toward a practise of decolonization*. BriarPatch.

Wallace, R. (2011). Power, practice and a critical pedagogy for non-Indigenous allies. *The Canadian Journal of Native Studies, 31*(2), 155–72, 189.

Weaver, S. (1993). The Hawthorn report: Its use in the making of Canadian Indian policy. In N. Dyck & J. Waldram (Eds.), *Anthropology, public policy and native peoples in Canada,* (pp. 75–97). McGill-Queen's University Press.

White, J., Wingert, S., Beavon, D.J., & Maxim, P. (2007a). *Aboriginal policy research: Moving forward, making a difference* (Vol. IV). Thompson Educational Publishing.

White, J., Beavon, D., & Spence, N. (2007b). *Aboriginal well-being: Canada's continuing challenge*. Thompson Educational Publishing.

White, J., & Maxim, P. (2007c). Community well-being: A comparable communities analysis. In J. White, D. Beavon, & N. Spence (Eds.), *Aboriginal well-being: Canada's continuing challenge*. Thompson Educational Publishing.

White, J., Maxim, P., & Whitehead, P. (2000) Social capital, social cohesion and population outcomes in Canada's First Nations communities. *PSC Discussion Papers Series, 14*(7), Article 1. Retrieved from http://ir.lib.uwo.ca/pscpapers/vol14/iss7/1

White, J., Peters, J., Dinsdale, J., & Beavon. D. (2009). *Aboriginal policy research: Learning, technology and spirituality* (Vol VI). Thompson Educational Publishing.

Whitley, R., & McKenzie, K. (2005). Social capital and psychiatry: Review of the literature. *Harvard Review of Psychiatry 13*(2), 71–84.

Wilkes, R. (2015). Indigenous resistance in comparative perspective: An overview with an autobiographical research critique. In E. Coburn (Ed.), *More will sing their way to freedom: Indigenous resistance and resurgence* (pp. 109–26). Fernwood Publishing.

Wilson, K., & Rosenberg, M. (2002). Exploring the determinants of health for First Nations peoples in Canada: Can existing frameworks accommodate traditional activities? *Social Science & Medicine, 55*(11), 2017–31.

Wilson, S. (2008). *Research is ceremony: Indigenous research methods*. Fernwood Publishing.

Wingert, S. (2011). The social distribution of distress and well-being in the Canadian Aboriginal population living off reserve. *The International Indigenous Policy Journal, 2*(1).

Woolcock, M. (2001). The place of social capital in understanding social and economic outcomes. *Canadian Journal of Policy Research, 2*(1), 11–17.

World Health Organization. (2006). *1948 Constitution of the World Health Organization*. Retrieved from http://apps.who.int/gb/bd/PDF/bd48/basic-documents-48th-edition-en.pdf#page=7

World Health Organization. (2020, October 12). *Coronavirus disease (COVID-19)*. Retrieved from https://www.who.int/emergencies/diseases/novel -coronavirus-2019/question-and-answers-hub/q-a-detail/coronavirus -disease-covid-19

Yin, R. (2003). *Case study research: Design and methods* (3rd ed.). Sage.

Yin, R. (2014). *Case study research: Design and methods* (5th ed.). Sage.

Index